MW00607429

AN UNFORTUNATE COINCIDENCE

AN UNFORTUNATE COINCIDENCE

A Mother's Life inside the Autism Controversy

Julie Obradovic

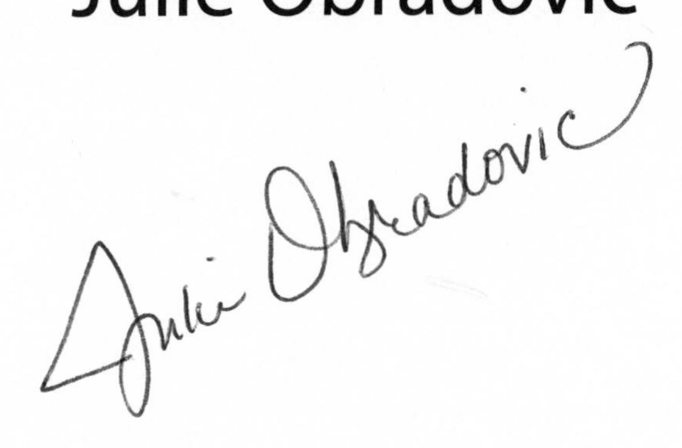

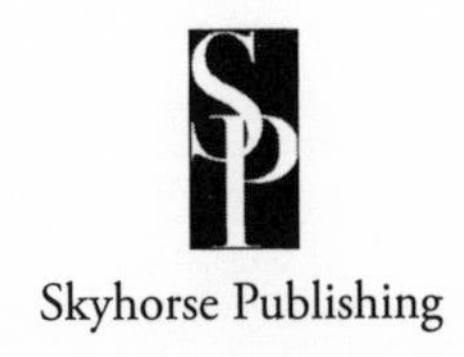

Skyhorse Publishing

Skyhorse Publishing books may be purchased in bulk at special discounts for sales promotion, corporate gifts, fund-raising, or educational purposes. Special editions can also be created to specifications. For details, contact the Special Sales Department, Skyhorse Publishing, 307 West 36th Street, 11th Floor, New York, NY 10018 or info@skyhorsepublishing.com.

Skyhorse® and Skyhorse Publishing® are registered trademarks of Skyhorse Publishing, Inc.®, a Delaware corporation.

Visit our website at www.skyhorsepublishing.com.

10 9 8 7 6 5 4 3 2 1

Library of Congress Cataloging-in-Publication Data is available on file.

Cover design by Rain Saukas
Cover photo: iStockphoto

Print ISBN: 978-1-5107-0462-6
Ebook ISBN: 978-1-5107-0463-3

Printed in the United States of America

For E.M.M.A.

CONTENTS

Introduction ix

Prologue xv

Part I: The Descent

Chapter 1: Vision—This Time, I'm Going to Get It Right 3

Chapter 2: Regression—Something's Wrong 17

Chapter 3: Suspicion—A Moment of Weakness 33

Chapter 4: Confirmation—Sometimes When We're Disappointed . . . 53

Part II: The Decisions

Chapter 5: Panic—Getting Away 71

Chapter 6: Investigation—There's a Book? 77

Chapter 7: Treatment—Blood on My Hands 95

Chapter 8: Recovery—Why Do Elephants Eat Grass? 109

Part III: The Resistance

Chapter 9: Activism—An Unfortunate Coincidence 125

Chapter 10: Anger—A Vaccine for Autism, or Something Like It 141

Chapter 11: Opposition—Organized Medicine Strikes Back 159

Chapter 12: Devastation—When Later Came 173

Part IV: The Result

Chapter 13: Acceptance—Take a Walk 193

Chapter 14: Horror—Who Killed Alex Spourdalakis? 205

Chapter 15: Revolt—The Consequence of Coincidence 217

Chapter 16: Testimony—Let the Science, and the Mothers, Speak 233

Epilogue 253

Acknowledgments 259

INTRODUCTION

I wanted a simple life. I planned on teaching high school for thirty-plus years at the same school in a nice suburb where I would get married, raise children, and vacation at my parents' lake house or travel during my summers off.

Never in my wildest dreams did I anticipate becoming involved in, nor did I want to become involved in, one of the biggest medical controversies in history. Never did I anticipate what the last twelve years of my life would entail, from blogging, to working for a documentary, to appearing on television, to testifying before Senate committees, to even working for Robert F. Kennedy, Jr. And never, ever did I imagine I would be able to tell the story in a book.

To be sure, what you're about to read is only my story and my opinion, based on the evidence I gathered, about how and why it happened, and later, what I chose to do about it. It's an explanation, not a thesis.

As I resent other people telling me how I should feel about my daughter and her autism, I know others feel the same. Under no circumstance should anyone take this account as the experience of everyone who has a child with autism or everyone who has autism.

If you love that your child or you yourself are on the spectrum, I think that's wonderful. I am not advocating discounting anyone or telling anyone how to feel.

But our experience was very different, and now that we are entering an era of autism acceptance, where the move to embrace it as a mental difference, not a medical disability, is gaining traction, I feel obligated to tell another side of the story. For us, autism was a devastating, frightening, mysterious journey into physical dysfunction, heartache, and struggle. One that I believe was entirely avoidable and preventable.

And although I can only speak for myself, I feel confident that this is also the experience of thousands of other parents, children, and families that I have met and befriended over the years. Our voices have been drowned out, however, our stories cast aside as anomalies best explained by coincidence, nothing more.

I don't believe there was anything coincidental about what happened to my daughter. In fact, I believe exactly what should have happened, actually happened. She and the other children like her are the canaries in the coal mine, showing us that too much medicine and too many toxins are combining to disable the vulnerable.

But because the focus of autism causation has centered on vaccines for so long—and rightfully so, I believe—other environmental co-factors have largely been ignored. In our case, I am not convinced it was only vaccines that pushed my daughter to autism's door. I truly believe that too many antibiotics, too many anti-inflammatories, toxic breast milk, toxic exposures in the womb, pollution, aluminum, and anesthesia all combined *with* too many vaccines to finally push her over the edge. However, I also believe none of that would have resulted in as much damage for her were it not for being exposed to mercury in the first place.

I am not alone in my belief that it is more than vaccines leading our children down a path to autism. Many mothers, especially mothers of children on the spectrum who have never vaccinated, believe the same. And antidepressants have recently become identified as a possible contributing factor as well as pesticides. It seems we all come to autism with similar ingredients, but the exposures, the doses, and the timing tend to vary.

What we have learned, however, is that by addressing these issues in our children, we can vastly improve their well-being. In some cases, like ours, children can recover substantially from the diagnosis.

This should be cause for celebration, but unfortunately it's not. The war over the paradigm of what autism is—either a lifelong, genetic, irreversible condition that's always been with us at a constant rate, or an environmentally caused, reversible condition that has exploded in epidemic proportions—has fractured the autism and medical communities, arguably to the point of paralysis. As a result, the vast majority of research remains in the genetic realm; the most often prescribed treatments are behavioral therapy and psychotropic medication.

We didn't choose to challenge the paradigm because we couldn't accept that our daughter might be genetically flawed—an insulting claim often made about parents like us who choose to treat autism as a medical condition, not a genetic one. We chose to do so because that's what our daughter, through her medical history and her medical tests, showed us was wrong. We felt we had a responsibility to rule out anything at the root of her autism that could help her feel better, and yes, perhaps, recover. We make no apologies for that.

However, at no point in time did we do so without the guidance of a medical doctor. Although I briefly mention some of the interventions we tried, I have purposefully not gone into detail about our protocol. Nothing in this book should be taken as medical advice of any kind.

As I mentioned, it's just a story. It's the real story of the parents so commonly demonized these days as conspiracy-theory, anti-science nutjobs that selfishly don't care if the world explodes in infectious disease with their "anti-vaccine" message. That's the popular narrative, at least. Parents like me have been dehumanized and discounted, mischaracterized and stereotyped as reckless perpetrators of a medical myth to be outcast and dismissed. Unfortunately, the mainstream narrative is the actual myth. We have much to teach the world.

Moreover, other books in the past few years have claimed to tell the true story of the vaccine autism controversy, to significant acclaim and reward, even though an outsider has written them. I don't believe that calling an unaffected person's version of events the "true story" is fair.

This is the true story of the vaccine autism controversy from someone who *lived* it. And even that's not an accurate description. It's about so much more than vaccines and autism.

This is really a story about love, hope, heartbreak, success, failure, intuition, abandonment, missed opportunity, medical orthodoxy, bullies, and the impact of historical misogyny, scientific and government corruption, eroding parental rights, and government overreach in our children's lives. Vaccines just happened to be the vehicle that exposes the underlying issues.

To be sure, the mainstream media and medical community say none of what I'm going to tell you actually happened in the way I am going to present it. It's all been an unfortunate coincidence, they insist.

And although I'm finally at a place where I have come to accept that this is the way it may be viewed for some time, I thought it might be worthwhile to tell our side of the story so you could understand why we don't share that view. I'm tired of being criticized and called names for challenging the default position. So are my friends.

Intending the book to be part memoir, part defense of parents, I organized it into four parts: Part I, "The Descent," captures the regression of our child into autism; Part II, "The Decisions," captures the decisions we made regarding how to move forward after the diagnosis; Part III, "The Resistance,"captures the pushback parents began experiencing from organized medicine by the end of the decade; and Part IV, "The Result," captures where we are today and why I believe that is where we are.

Overall, the book is in chronological order from approximately 1998 to 2016, although in some instances, I have flashed back or forward if necessary. For the protection of my family, friends, colleagues, and physicians, names, genders, and locations have sometimes been changed.

Is autism really a long line of unfortunate coincidences, as the mainstream view wants us to believe? Or is it tragically unfortunate, but not the least bit coincidental, after all? I know what I have lived, as well as what I believe.

You decide.

PROLOGUE

From what I remember, I enjoyed the hospital. At night, after my parents left, another girl on the floor and I would ride our wheelchairs up and down the aisles. We would race, circle around, and see how far we could roll with one giant push. It made the experience much less scary.

I was only there for two days, but I can still remember my gown, the room, and the beautiful white barrettes my uncle's fiancée gave me. I loved them and was heartbroken when I lost them years later.

I knew why I had been brought to the hospital but not why I had to stay. The day before, an overcast and dreary April afternoon, I asked my mom if I could ride my bike to my friend's house. We had just moved to a suburb of Chicago. I barely knew anyone but had made a new friend. After getting home from kindergarten, I wanted to play.

Amy's house was only a handful away from mine, but it was at the top of a hill. From there, you could see the coal-burning plant five miles directly to the west. Riding up it required a lot of effort for someone who had only recently gotten rid of her training wheels. I made it, rang the bell, and was disappointed to learn she was taking a nap.

"Maybe tomorrow," her mom said with a smile.

I got back on my new powder-blue bike with the banana seat and white plastic basket with a daisy and headed home. Only this time, I had to ride down the hill. I had no experience doing such a thing, as there were no hills in my old neighborhood.

I started gaining speed almost immediately. The cracks on the sidewalk went by faster and faster, and soon I realized I was no longer in charge of the pedals beneath my feet. I panicked and held on tightly. It was then I remembered the bump in the road, the one caused by the sidewalk sinking several inches lower than the curb. I knew when I hit it, I would likely pop in the air and fall.

Regardless, I couldn't stop myself. The bike approached at alarming speed, and just like I predicted, running into the bump launched me into the air. I flew over the handlebars and landed flat on my back in the middle of the street. I don't remember anything after that for about the next hour.

I was lying on my bed with the shades pulled, my mom sitting next to me, not allowing me to go to sleep. She kept asking me questions, sitting me up, and singing songs with me. We talked for a little while until I finally felt sick and threw up. Immediately thereafter, we rode in our yellow paneled station wagon to the emergency room, where I was diagnosed with a concussion and admitted for a two-night stay for observation.

My parents were constantly by my side, but once in a while there was a lapse. I would then be alone in my hospital room with my coloring books, the TV remote, my stuffed animal, and my cool bed, which I couldn't believe had the ability to go up and down like it did. The place seemed magical.

During one of those times, a nurse delivered my lunch. Under the plate cover I expected to find something close to what I'd gotten the day before: peanut butter and jelly on white bread, some fruit, and something else.

But this day, I had no such luck. Staring back at me to my horror was an awful sight: a tuna-fish sandwich on wheat. I made the face of a six-year-old staring at food she couldn't possibly contemplate eating and put the lid back on. I thanked the person who brought it and went back to my coloring.

Some time passed before my mom returned to find my meal untouched. Upon investigating, she knew the reason. Although I wasn't a picky child, there were a few things I would absolutely never eat: pot roast and fish.

"I hate fish," I reminded her matter-of-factly.

The story was told many times throughout my childhood, especially whenever someone would serve fish. Sometimes my parents would tell it, and sometimes I would tell it. When I met my husband's family, big seafood eaters, I used it to explain the depths with which I despised it. Everyone who knew me knew I didn't eat fish, and especially not tuna.

And I didn't. Ever. At least not until June 2001. And then I ate it a couple of times a week . . . for several weeks . . . while breastfeeding.

PART I

THE DESCENT

Chapter 1

Vision—This Time, I'm Going to Get It Right

The pizza tasted like crap. It added to the already miserable experience I was having on my own in Alaska. I was starving after finishing my first marathon, and I really wanted to eat the whole thing. I just couldn't.

I was also in pain. Training in the Midwest for over a year, I ran almost exclusively on flat land. Occasionally, I would meet a nasty hill, but rarely.

Alaska was nothing like home, and neither was the marathon. I had wanted to run the Chicago marathon the previous fall, but I trained too hard and hurt myself. That marathon, always held in October, had to pass without me.

When I got better, I was still in the best shape of my life. I was also in the best place of my life. I had finished college the year before with a degree in teaching high school Spanish. I even got a job offer at the first school where I interviewed.

It was close to my parents' home, where I still lived while saving money. Worried I might not have another offer, I took it, but deep inside, I knew it wasn't right for me. Something just didn't feel right. My excitement became overshadowed by anxiety.

As I predicted, that year wasn't my favorite. In addition to hurting my foot, I quickly learned that my instinct was right. I resigned after a very unhappy experience at the end of the school year. It was the first time as an adult I ignored my intuition to my own serious detriment. Unfortunately, it would not even come close to being the last.

I sank into a slight depression that year and started relying more on my boyfriend, Mike, to make me feel better. I became needy and clingy, and whereas only a few months earlier I couldn't have cared less about getting married, now I suddenly found myself obsessed with the thought. It was all I could think about to escape my sadness.

I began to fantasize about our life together, where we would live, and how many children we would have. I would think about the kind of mom I would be, how I would raise our kids, what was important to me, and what they would look like.

This I knew for sure. Between the two of us, both honor students, outgoing, athletic, college grads, our children would be amazing. I wanted five of them. That any of them would ever have a health problem never crossed my mind.

I got to Alaska after a very long, lonely plane ride. Most of the people on the trip had either trained together or knew one another. I knew no one and spent most of my time walking around the campus where we stayed, taking in the fresh air.

I also slept a lot. For at least the week prior, I had been exhausted. It was a different kind of exhaustion though, one where I could flop down face first on my bed and be asleep within moments. When my parents asked why I was so tired all of a sudden, I reassured them, as I did myself, that it was all the running I was doing.

The last few weeks of training were intense, I told them. I had a twenty-miler on a Saturday, came home, and slept until Sunday. I would knock out thirteen miles on a Wednesday. I was on pace to finish in less than four hours, maybe much less, and I was determined I would. All of this, I convinced myself, was why I was so tired. It was also why I missed my period.

I was in the middle of these thoughts as I stared at the pizza I had waited over an hour to be delivered. I was irritated, and I was in pain. At one point, unexpectedly changing terrain, crossing over the dirt trail in the mountains to the concrete highway alongside it, I fractured my foot. I didn't know that yet and somehow finished the race. Now, I realized I had really screwed it up by running through the pain.

To break the silence, the boredom, the irritation, and the worry, I called my parents, as I said I would. Yes, I finished the race, in just a little over four hours, I boasted.

But that was a lie. I actually finished in well over five. Even though I thought it was highly unlikely, and that I would give it a few more weeks before confirming with my doctor, I worried dearly that if I were pregnant, I could be hurting the baby. I decided to run the race, but very, very slowly just in case.

False start

We decided to get legally married a few months before our son was born. And that fall, after I got a new teaching position, we bought a small Cape Cod house in the suburbs.

I began home improvement projects immediately—first, our son's nursery. It had always weighed heavily on me that I did not welcome him into our lives prepared. I was relieved to finally give him the stability I so desperately desired, but even that was short-lived. Six months after moving in, due to a serious issue with a neighbor, we were forced to move.

By then, all I wanted to do was find a place to settle down, relax, enjoy our son, and have another baby when the time was right. Not far from my childhood home, to be close to my parents, we purchased a house much like the one where I had grown up. Finally, we could start our lives, I sighed. It was May 1999.

Within a year, we had a good routine. It was the first time I could measure how long it would take to get through something stressful as an adult. A year it seemed; everything would be over in a year. And in this case, it was.

I loved my new job, and even though I hated leaving my baby boy, he was in the wonderful hands of his grandmothers. Both generously offered to watch him while I taught. By the spring of the following year, I was ready to give him a sibling. In June 2000, I got pregnant with my second child. And this time, I vowed, it would be different.

I didn't find out the sex with my first pregnancy. I would now, I decided. I didn't have the nursery done for my son. This time, it would be done well ahead of time. With him, I didn't know what I was doing. This time, I would be perfect.

Everything about this pregnancy and birth would be different, I assured myself. I was ready for this one. We had our home. We had good jobs. We had all of the baby products, and they were well researched and ready to go. We even had a minivan.

In my mind, we were as prepared as anyone could be.

It's a girl!

Emma was born in late March. The birth was quiet and easy. There was no time for an epidural—the time between my first labor pain and her birth was no more than six hours. Unlike my son, who even with an epidural left me feeling like I had been run over by a truck, I felt no pain after my daughter's birth. I went home within less than forty-eight hours feeling fabulous.

I was, however, on medication. I was given an antibiotic prior to delivery because I tested positive for Group B streptococcus. She, too, was on an antibiotic. Although she hadn't aspirated any, meconium was detected in her bag of water. Even so, she was given a clean bill of health.

In the hospital, before we left, I believe she received two injections, a hepatitis B vaccine and vitamin K shot. To my recollection, I was not asked about either. I just saw the little adhesive bandages afterward, asked what they were for, and really thought nothing of it. In fact, I was actually glad I hadn't been privy to the procedure. I never wanted to be a part of anything that could hurt my children, even if it were for their own good.

Instead, I just gushed over her beauty. Emma was a breathtaking little baby. Her coloring, her skin, and her face were beautiful. She looked like an angel, and she acted like one too. She cried appropriately, but hardly ever, sleeping comfortably and quietly. She also latched on to my breast with no trouble.

I held her in awe, recognizing right away that she looked exactly like my husband's sister. I also thought that she looked little. My son had weighed almost eight pounds, and he looked bigger. He had been plump. Emma was not. She was an inch longer than he had been and a full pound lighter. I instantly felt guilty that she didn't have enough fat on her.

I had gone to great lengths to control my weight with her pregnancy. At several months pregnant, I barely looked pregnant, and I wore that like a badge of honor. The message from our culture was clear—even if you were a mother, you didn't want to look like one. We want women to look like they can have babies; we just don't actually want them to change their bodies to have them. It was not unusual to see celebrities on the cover of magazines in bikinis weeks after giving birth. It still isn't.

And so guilt was something I was already feeling not a day into her birth. But not even an hour into it, I felt something entirely different. I felt concerned. I knew within moments of first looking at her in the incubator that something would go wrong with this child.

It hit me like a flash of lightning. I can't describe it other than a deep, primal, inexplicable knowing. From her tiny frame to the way she looked in the warming bed, something in me knew, someday, somehow, some way, this child would get sick. It scared the hell out of me.

Like I do with most instincts I have that I don't want to have, I talked myself out of it. I entertained the thought just long enough to realize what I felt, and then shook my head side to side as if to fling it away. It was just nerves, I lied to myself, a normal feeling many mothers have about their children. It was natural to feel that way, I determined.

But I knew better. I did not feel that way with her brother, not once. Not even when he developed colic, thrush, and acidic diarrhea. I never worried anything was wrong with him, except for maybe having my lazy eye.

I had to wear a patch as child because of it, so I always looked at my son's eyes very carefully. I would do the same with Emma for years; it would be the first way I ever knew for sure she had autism.

In less than forty-eight hours, we packed our things and headed home. As soon as we got settled, I went into my bathroom and weighed myself. I was curious how much weight you lost right after you had a baby.

Thirteen pounds was the answer. I stared at myself with pride. I looked good and I felt good, unlike last time. My stomach was already going down. I wasn't the least bit swollen. Whatever I had done, I had done something right, I decided.

I got out my pregnancy bible, *What to Expect When You're Expecting*, where I had tracked my weekly weight gain, and entered my "after birth" weight. Now I would track my weekly weight loss.

"Only twenty-two more pounds to go," I said to myself with a smile.

It was six weeks until my sister-in-law's wedding, when I had to fit into a bridesmaid's dress, and only three months after that until my cousin's wedding in August. I was sure I could lose the baby weight by August and as determined that I would as I had been to finish that marathon in Alaska.

Getting my body back

On April 14, 2001, a little over two weeks after Emma was born, I went to my parents' house to watch the Masters Tournament with my dad, a tradition. I came over with Emma, wearing a pair of size eight jeans and a t-shirt from a race I ran while training for the marathon.

I know this because I have pictures of us. You could hardly tell I had a baby, and Emma was still teeny tiny in a beautiful pink cotton outfit. I placed a blanket on the ground for her to lie on while we watched TV.

While taking pictures of her, I noticed a red dot in the middle of her cheek. It looked like a pimple, but it wasn't. At first, I wondered if I had scratched her or if she had scratched herself, but it clearly wasn't a scratch. It was just a bump, a bright, red, random bump. For the second time, my instinct told me something was wrong. For the second time, I ignored it.

Later that day, my dad and I talked about diet and exercise. He left a popular fitness book that he found some success with on the table for me. I had told him about my plan to get fit by the end of summer, and that I was sick of just running, which is why he suggested it. I took it home and read it in detail that night.

Not long into it, however, I became very disappointed. The program called for several small meals a day, all with some form of protein. There were bars and shakes that you could buy, but even then, you needed to eat real food most of the time. The options for fruits and vegetables were unlimited, but the choices for protein were not—mostly eggs, chicken breast, or fish.

I almost gave the book back then. There was not a chance I was going to eat fish for several weeks. I hated fish, and I had never eaten it in my entire life. Still, the idea of looking great by August lingered in my mind. Maybe I could stomach it for a few weeks, I persuaded myself. Besides, everyone knew fish was really good for you.

I was breastfeeding at that time, but not exclusively. A breast infection that required another round of antibiotics curbed my success. I worried that Emma had been exposed to two rounds of antibiotics through me in less than the first few months of her life, not to mention the ones she had been given at birth, and I decided to wean her early. Within three months, she was more bottle fed than breastfed, and by six months of age, I had stopped breastfeeding entirely.

Still, I knew I needed to wait six weeks to start dieting or exercising. Given the great shape I was in and that I felt fine, I was given the green light to do so moderately by my doctor when the time came.

As the weeks passed and I anxiously awaited the opportunity to start my program, Emma's red dot morphed into many, many more. Over the course of a month, it went on to cover her entire face. At its worst, it looked like someone had burned her, like her cheeks had been scalded. I was horrified, as I had never seen anything like it.

The doctors told me they weren't sure what it was, but that it was probably contact dermatitis, warning me not to wash her with any harsh chemicals. I assured them I had not, let alone on her face, but they did not offer any other explanation.

I looked for information about pediatric rashes in the reference books I had and came up with a few possibilities, but none of them quite matched what she had. It wasn't any of the typical ones you might expect to find in a two-month-old. (And this was almost two years before I even knew Google existed. I never used the Internet to find medical information at that time.)

But no matter what the doctors said, I just knew it was not caused by something external. Her body was rejecting something, reacting to something internally. For years, I didn't think about it again, until one day I gasped at a photo being shared on the Internet of an infant with the exact same rash lying in a hospital bed.

According to his parents, he had a reaction to his hepatitis B vaccine . . . and died.

Is that safe?

The first wedding passed, and the following week, I began my fitness program. I set up a weight system in the basement; organized a binder with places to document my workouts, my diet, and my progress; and put the book of how to do the exercises with it for easy access. For several weeks, I managed to eat only chicken and eggs for my protein, but I soon became sick of them. I would have to find a way to eat some tuna, I decided.

I sent Mike to the store to buy it since I couldn't stomach the thought. He came back with at least a dozen cans that emphasized the combination of protein and good fatty acids that made tuna a responsible nutritional choice. The cans did not mention, however, the new FDA warning from a few months prior.

According to the *New York Times*, who reported on the topic on January 13, 2001, "Pregnant women and those who might become pregnant should not eat shark, swordfish, king mackerel or tilefish, because they could contain enough mercury to hurt an unborn baby's developing brain, the government has warned. In issuing the warning on Friday, the Food and Drug Administration rejected calls to also put tuna on the list, saying the other fish contain far more mercury than tuna does."

And so, nowhere on the can was mercury mentioned. Nowhere was it advertised on grocery store shelves, like it is for alcohol or tobacco, that eating tuna or other big fish can be dangerous and should be limited while one is pregnant or nursing.

Nowhere was it mentioned that even though the Environmental Protection Agency believes the safe level of exposure to mercury for anyone should be no more than 0.1 micrograms per day, according to a report in *Men's Health* magazine, the average five-ounce can of chunk light tuna contains 18.11 micrograms, and the average can of albacore tuna contains 49.53 micrograms.

I had no idea that by eating one can of tuna once or twice a week for several weeks, I possibly consumed anywhere from 150 micrograms of methyl mercury to over 400 micrograms, depending on what type of tuna I had eaten. (We do not know for sure, but we are almost certain it was chunk light tuna.) And I had no idea I was feeding some of that to my baby.

Nowhere at any point in my life had the danger of mercury ever been discussed. Absolutely no one, not even my doctors, had taught me or talked to me about the dangers of mercury . . . except for my best friend.

A little over a month into the program, we shared one of our lengthy phone conversations. During that time, I mentioned the workouts and what I was eating. She paused and asked me if that was okay, as she had recently heard it was bad for pregnant women to eat big fish.

I wasn't pregnant, I assured her, laughing it off. And I wasn't eating a big fish, either, I thought. She knew that, but said it had something to do with mercury. She didn't know why there was mercury or what it could do, only that it was bad. The FDA had recently said so, she insisted.

Later that day, I went upstairs to the nursery where I took out my pregnancy and baby bibles once more just to check that I hadn't missed something important: The American Academy of Pediatrics' *Caring for Your Baby and Young Child: Birth to Age 5* by Steven Shelov, MD, the 1994 edition, and *What to Expect When You're Expecting* by Arlene Eisenberg, Heidi Murkoff, and Sandee Hathaway, the 1996 edition. It seemed highly unlikely I had done anything dangerous, but I wanted to be sure.

The first book did not have the words *mercury* or *fish* in it at all. Nowhere in over 600 pages of information were those words mentioned. The second book, however, did have them, but claimed eating a few cans of tuna a week during pregnancy was fine.

On page 130, it read, "As a general rule, [pregnant women] should also skip freshwater fish caught in polluted lakes and rivers (most are). It's also recommended that they limit intake of swordfish, fresh tuna, and shark (all high in mercury) to no more than one serving per month (though because levels are lower in canned tuna, a couple of cans a week are okay)."

Seeing that the first book didn't mention it, and that the second book said a few cans a week during pregnancy was okay, I breathed a sigh of relief. I thought, *this can't be that bad.* If it were, obviously it would have been not only common knowledge, but also labeled and discussed prominently.

There would be warning labels for mercury, screening tools, and laws, I reasoned, just like there were for lead. Lead, everyone my age knew, was extremely toxic for a child. We even had to fill out a questionnaire about it when we bought a house and at the pediatrician's office. No one ever talked about mercury being the same or worse. No one ever asked about our exposure to it or screened us for it, either.

The feeling that I may have done something horrible, however, gnawed at me. I sat in the glider chair holding the books to my chest, contemplating calling her doctor just to make sure I hadn't.

But clearly, I reminded myself, I couldn't have. It's not on the can. It's not on the shelves. It's not in the book. No one talks about this. My doctor never said a word. My husband didn't know. My father didn't know.

Even my best friend wasn't sure why you shouldn't eat fish while pregnant, only that you shouldn't. Plus, it was shark and swordfish I had to avoid, the book said. Canned tuna was fine, it claimed. And I'm not pregnant, I kept telling myself. *I'm not pregnant.* Emma was almost three months old, and I was only breastfeeding her half of the time, anyway.

I slowly walked downstairs and gently picked up the phone from the wall. In the family room below, I could see her sleeping peacefully in her swing, where I left her. Besides the rash, which I knew they didn't have any idea about anyway, she was perfect. Her coloring, her sleep, her poops, her development, and her disposition were all perfect. I took a deep breath and told myself to relax. Everything was fine. I was overreacting, something I have often been accused of.

I put the phone back on the hook and walked over to the pantry. There I angrily pushed all of the remaining cans to the back, double-checking that they didn't have a warning I missed somewhere. Nope, they didn't. I relaxed even more, now irritated more than anything. I even got mad at my friend for making me worry.

Just to be safe, I decided I would never eat it again. I was aggravated that I hadn't trusted my taste buds or my gut. I knew there was a reason I always hated fish, and I was disgusted that the only time I ever ate it in my entire life was a few times a week for a little over a month while breastfeeding my daughter.

What were the chances of that?

Within a month, the rash cleared. Emma was a healthy, vibrant, laughing little angel who was engaged and all smiles, a breeze to take care of, and an easy sleeper to boot. The summer got underway with great joy.

I took her for her three-month photos at the Sears studio, like I had done with her brother, and proudly shared them with the family. She could roll over and firmly hold her head, and her hair was finally coming in. Her perfectly sized round head, the nicest shaped baby head I had ever seen, looked beautiful in the one photo I took without a hat.

I stared at the gorgeous photo for months, framing it to display in our entry hall. My sister-in-law claimed that my daughter oozed joy and light in it, and every day I looked at it proudly and carefully, thinking the same.

My daughter was perfect. And thankfully, in spite of my worries, so were her eyes. There was no sign of anything wrong with her vision (or mine for her future), as they beamed back at me happily.

Chapter 2

Regression—Something's Wrong

On September 29, 2001, I entered Emma's room to get her from her nap. Through the baby monitor, I could hear she was ready to get up. I gently opened the door and greeted her with a soft voice.

I glanced in the crib where she lay and went to the window to open the shade and let in some light. I carefully lifted it to not overwhelm her eyes and smiled as I leaned over to pick her up. Then I noticed something coming out of her left ear: a pool of gooey liquid the color of earwax.

I looked at her horrified with two instantaneous thoughts. One, something was very wrong, and two, why wasn't she crying?

Immediately, I called her pediatrician for some clarification. No, she hadn't been cranky or miserable. No, she didn't feel warm or have a fever. And no, she didn't appear to be upset. They thought that was odd, as did I, and told me to come right in. I packed up and left.

At the office, I was informed she had a severe ear infection that had caused her eardrum to burst. I started to tear up at the thought, unable to imagine how much that must have hurt. I felt like a terrible mother, but more so, terribly worried. The whole thing was just odd.

Her brother never had an ear infection, so I had no experience with them. In my very naïve way, I chalked that up to my superior parenting. Several people I knew with children his age were constantly battling ear infections, and their kids were on antibiotics all the time. I assumed it was because they were in day care or because they didn't eat very nutritious food. That was another thing I heard about quite a bit lately—picky eaters. My son was no such thing, nor did he attend day care.

But neither did Emma. My mother and mother-in-law were still generously caring for the kids as I continued to teach that year. Although I was exposed to germs at school, such exposure was no different for her than it was for her brother. And he was never sick. Neither was Mike, nor was I.

The doctor asked me again about her symptoms for the few days prior. I repeated that there was nothing unusual. She was sleeping well, eating well, and seemed happy. This had been a very strange turn of events.

It was then I had a terrible thought. What if she couldn't feel it? Was it possible she didn't? Was her sense of pain not functioning normally? I once saw a television special about people who had that problem. I decided to ask.

The doctor turned slightly on his stool to face me, halfway looking up from the chart where he was writing something. In a quiet voice, with a tone that was gentle but clearly communicated he thought I was an idiot for suggesting such a thing, he responded, "No, it's not possible she didn't feel it. You might just need to pay a little bit better attention to your child."

And with that, he turned back to his folder.

I couldn't breathe for a second. The air left my lungs; I felt virtually punched in the gut. I had always loved this doctor, but in an instant, I hated him. He was blaming me. I was the reason this baby burst an eardrum. I was the one who wasn't paying attention. And I was the reason she was suffering. Not only that, he thought I was making up excuses for my bad mothering.

I didn't say a word the rest of the time. He gave me a prescription for an antibiotic and told me to come back in two weeks to make sure the infection cleared and the eardrum healed. We gathered our things and left; I felt guilty, embarrassed, and was slowly becoming enraged.

By the time I got home, I was furious. I thought about all of the things I wished I said to that doctor while imagining the scene playing out differently.

Pay attention to your child? Pay attention to your child! Who the hell do you think you are? You want to come to my house and verify how much I pay attention to this child? You want to see the books I read to her every day, the stroller I walk her in, and the photos I take constantly?

You want me to videotape the nightly bath routine we have and the personalized nursery rhyme that I made up just for her? Would you like to see her two closets full of clothes given to her by the enormous, loving family and circle of friends she is attended to and adored by?

Would you like to check your records and see that I haven't missed a single appointment to date? That when it says to be there at two months, I actually try to get there on that exact date, and any delay is due to your office not having availability?

Have you forgotten we were just in there two weeks ago on September 10, 2001, to receive her second series of vaccines? Where she received the DTaP, pneumococcal, polio, and Hib/hep B shots at the same time? Because I remember being there. It was the day before the world turned upside down. Life was one way that Monday, and a completely different way by the end of Tuesday.

Pay attention to your child! Go fuck yourself.

When I get angry or upset, I talk to myself out loud. I can have whole conversations with nobody, just to hear my voice and vent. It is in those conversations I have the courage to say what I don't otherwise.

Suddenly, thinking about the September 10 appointment gave me pause. I remembered something. Just like her June 5 appointment, where she received the same vaccines as September 10, I loaded her up on Tylenol before I left. One of my closest friends was in medical school at the time, and we just so happened to be on the phone the morning of her two-month checkup.

"Load her up on Tylenol before you go," she insisted. "It will help the pain if she's got some in her system already before she gets the shots."

I followed her advice. I did the same on September 10. But then I remembered something I had forgotten about until then. After her June 5 shots, she developed a very hard lump on her leg at the injection site.

It wasn't a little lump either; it was big goose-egg type of lump, raised, hard, and warm to the touch. It took weeks to go away. I also remembered that she developed very acidic poops at that time. Her little butt had gotten raw from diaper rash.

For a few moments, I wondered if any of that had anything to do with this ear infection. After thinking about it, however, I changed my mind. How could vaccines have anything to do with an ear infection? They couldn't, I decided. But still, it seemed odd. There was a pattern developing.

She got a shot while on antibiotics in the hospital, and a rash developed all over her face shortly after that. She got four shots for eight diseases while on Tylenol and developed a lump on her leg and acidic diarrhea. And now she got the same four shots for eight diseases while on Tylenol and had an ear infection three weeks later. And not just any ear infection, a serious ear infection. One, I was fairly convinced, she really didn't even feel.

I walked over to the closet and took out my baby bibles again. I looked up vaccine reactions, but there weren't any listed other than the same ones I had been warned about, possible low-grade fever, swelling at the injection site, and irritability. Even the two-sided, poorly copied sheet from the CDC they gave me at the doctor's office that was folded in the bottom of my diaper bag didn't mention much.

I put the books away, reassured again that the lack of information they shared was proof positive there was nothing to what I was thinking, and grabbed her baby book. There were a few pages for medical visits, vaccinations, and first teeth that I had been filling out, but instead, I went to the back cover where there was plenty of space.

On the top of the page I wrote the dates of the doctor visits, and under them the dates of the strange medical problems appearing. I made sure to write very small. Somehow I knew I was going to need that whole page.

Another, and another, and another

The ear infection cleared, but getting Emma to take medicine was an experience I would have rather never had. The amoxicillin was dyed bright pink, and she really didn't care for it. We would syringe it down her throat while trying not to gag her, holding her tilted backward in our arms, per the nurse's instructions, so that she would have to swallow. Even then, she would trick us and, right when we thought we were safe, would sit up and spit it out. I couldn't tell you how many bibs and outfits were ruined.

It was stressful, and I prayed that we would never have to use any kind of medication again. This was not a cooperative child when it came to medicine. Unfortunately, however, that prayer was not answered.

She got another ear infection in the same ear on November 30, six weeks to the day after her six-month shots on October 23. It was also exactly two months since the first one. In spite of my concern, she was given another ten days of amoxicillin.

The pattern continued for the next two years. On December 27, only two weeks off of her second round of antibiotics for her second ear infection, she was vaccinated again.

Three weeks later, she developed a serious respiratory infection, and on February 2, she was so sick that, as we waited in the doctor's examination room, her wheezing prompted a different doctor to burst into the room and put her on a nebulizer. He thought she might have the beginning stages of pneumonia. He also informed us she had not one more ear infection, but two. Both ears were severely infected.

This time, they gave us nebulizer treatments, and they changed the antibiotic to Augmentin. Augmentin, they warned, was rough on a baby's belly. She would have to have to something in her every time we dosed it. Whereas I hoped the change in medication would mean less stress in giving it to her, I was wrong. She hated the Augmentin even more.

Worse, it didn't work. Only ten days later, on February 13, we were back at the doctor's office. She was still very congested, struggling to breathe, and now had a fever of 102 with a scary cough. We were given more Augmentin anyway.

Driving to the doctor's office by then had become a major pain in the ass. The doctors I chose when my son was born reflected the location of the townhouse we first rented together. Getting there took over thirty minutes each way now.

For checkups, it didn't matter that they weren't close, but for this situation, I was having second thoughts. Not only weren't they close, they had also insulted me. More importantly, nothing they were doing was making her better.

At one point, they stopped having me come in to check whether the medication had actually cleared the ear infection. I no longer had any idea if she was getting new infections or if they were the same ones. And all the while, she was constantly on Motrin or Tylenol for pain.

In March 2002, after her third round of Augmentin for another double ear infection, she developed thrush in her mouth and a nasty vaginal yeast infection. Because her brother had thrush just shy of one month old, I knew right away what was wrong with Emma when I saw her inflamed gums and cheeks.

She was placed on an antifungal, and just like her brother, suffered from fluffy, bright yellow, nonstop diarrhea. If I didn't change her immediately, her delicate bottom would be raw with red patches.

The thrush in her mouth cleared, but the vaginal infection was more stubborn. As a woman, I knew how horrible yeast infections could be, and my heart ached for her. This poor kid was terribly ill all of the time.

Soon, new problems began emerging. She broke out in tender, red, inflamed patches of eczema on her ankles, behind her knees, and in her elbow creases. She developed dark circles under her eyes. She began drooling quite a bit, to the point where we always had to have a bib on her. And she didn't seem to be able to speak as much as her brother had been able to at her age.

Yet in spite of the fact that she was always on medication and suffering, she remained for the most part in a great mood. She smiled often, laughed a lot, and was still a very good baby.

But around nine months of age, after her second ear infection, I started to notice something more troublesome than the illnesses. Her body was changing. She seemed weaker. Whereas she could sit up on her own months earlier, now she no longer could really balance that well without a pillow propping her up or something supporting her.

And as crazy as it seemed, given it was winter and everyone got paler at that time, I swore she lost her coloring. Her rosy warm glow, that healthy vibrant coloring she had since birth, was gone. Emma was as white as a ghost.

Her head also appeared to swell. The beautiful round baby head she had was gone. Now she looked different. Her head looked huge to me.

She also never learned to crawl. Instead, she would push herself up with her arms and then log roll everywhere. Even more alarming was the way she would go from sitting to rolling. She would place her legs slightly out to the sides, lean forward, and then halfway down, then quickly fold her legs behind her. From that position, she would prop herself up with her arms and hands while on her belly and log roll to what she wanted.

It was the weirdest thing I had ever seen. People joked that she would be a great gymnast, but my grandmother, an Austrian immigrant, eighty-three years old at the time, a mother of three, aunt of many, and grandmother of eight, didn't like it. She would ask me about it to the point of me getting angry, and every time I insisted that the doctors told me everything was fine, would remark, "Doctors," shaking her head with a smirk. "Nobody ever listened to them until antibiotics. Now everybody thinks they're gods. I'm telling you, Julie Ann, something is wrong with that child."

The first birthday, 2002

Her first birthday passed, but it wasn't pleasant. Emma was recovering from another ear infection, just off another round of antibiotics, and her yeast infections were not gone. In her photos, she is pointing at her cake with a smile, but her little mouth is bright red. She also started drooling quite a bit around then, which we chalked up to the thrush.

And for the first time, as I looked more closely at our photographs of her party, I noticed her eyes didn't look right. There was something hazy about them, like she was looking through us, not at us. I convinced myself it was just the camera angle.

Three weeks later, on April 18, we were back in the doctor's office for yet another ear infection. By then, I had lost track of how many she had; perhaps this was yet another time that the one from weeks beforehand simply hadn't cleared. I begged to see if there were a different antibiotic, or whether there was a point to the antibiotics, as they clearly didn't seem to be helping.

The doctor put us back on amoxicillin anyway and sent us on our way, but not before asking if she was talking and meeting other developmental milestones. I had already shared with him what she was doing oddly, and he didn't express to me in any way that he was concerned.

I was told not every child crawled. And yes, she was talking a little. She had a few words and was pointing at things nicely. I even had the picture of her in my purse pointing at her birthday candle. And that very week, just shy of being thirteen months old, she learned to walk. The doctor seemed to feel she was fine.

On the way out, I asked the nurse to reschedule my twelve-month checkup, only five days from then. It seemed silly to come back in five days to basically answer the same questions. Besides, they were quite familiar with us by then, as we were in the office so often.

But the main reason I wanted to reschedule was that I knew that she was due for her next round of vaccinations. She hadn't had any since December, followed by the respiratory illness and double ear infection, and I was now convinced there was something to this.

Even if I were wrong, I still thought it made sense to wait. She would still be on antibiotics in five days. There was no way I was also vaccinating her while she was on them. The idea that you would make a baby's fragile immune system work harder on purpose seemed ridiculous.

I told the nurse my concerns, not even thinking for a second she wouldn't agree. I couldn't have been more wrong. The nurse, reminding me of the doctor after the first ear infection, stopped what she was doing to look at me.

"Don't change that appointment," she said seriously. "She is exactly the baby who needs to be up-to-date on her shots. It's because her immune system is so fragile we must make sure she is protected."

I sat in the chair with Emma on my lap once again feeling like the worst mother in the world. Clearly, I was an idiot. Every time I wanted to help this child, I seemed to want to do the wrong thing. I could only imagine what they had written about me in that file. *Ditzy mother with a dirty house who doesn't pay attention to her child.*

Beginning to question vaccines and us. Chronically sick kid. Keep an eye on this one.

We packed our stuff and left, and I kept the appointment as it was. We returned five days later on April 23, 2002, while she was still on her antibiotic. That day, she received her Hib/hep B and varicella vaccines.

Disney World

Over the course of the next six months, Emma suffered from at least four more ear infections. In June, we left her for one week to stay with my in-laws as we took a trip to Disney World with our son and my parents. She wouldn't remember, we reasoned, and being so sick all of the time, we worried about her on a plane around so many people. The nurse confirmed she was a vulnerable child. We left her back in Chicago.

When we returned, I couldn't wait to see her. In theory, leaving her behind had seemed like a good idea, but in reality, I regretted it. Plenty of people had their one-year-olds with them, and every time I saw them, I felt a pang of guilt and sadness. I rushed over to my mother-in-law's and scooped her out of bed with a giant hug.

While we were gathering her things to go home, my mother-in-law cautiously asked if I thought her hearing was all right. It was a legitimate question, I believed, given that the poor child had suffered from over ten ear infections in the past year. I told her I didn't know but had never been told there was a problem. She insisted I look into it.

"I'm calling her name, and she's not looking at me, Julie. It's like she doesn't even know I exist."

I made a note of it but tried not to think much about it. It made sense that she couldn't hear. That's all it was, I decided. All the while, the little voice I heard from the moment I looked at her in the incubator was growing louder.

"The doctors said she is fine," I would repeat to myself to drown it out. *The doctors said she is fine.*

The other birthday, 2002

In November that year, the day after our fifth anniversary, Mike turned thirty. I planned a surprise party for him, and in order to make it happen, my aunt, who was also my godmother, was kind enough to watch the kids.

We arrived home around 1:00 a.m., and right as we walked in the door, she appeared on the stairway looking like she had seen a ghost. Initially, I thought we just startled her, but I was wrong.

"I'm so glad you're home," she said nervously. "I was just about to call 911. Emma let out a scream a few minutes ago unlike anything I have ever heard. I seriously thought someone was stabbing her!"

As is sometimes the case for me when there is an urgent situation, I unexpectedly grew extremely calm. In nonemergency stressful situations, I panic easily. Put a bug on me, and you'll see a very over-reactive freak-out.

But in some emergencies, where life and death could be involved, the exact opposite happens. I don't fight or flee, but freeze. I become completely still, hyperaware of everything around me.

I can only describe it as an almost out-of-body experience. It had happened to me at least twice in my life by then, and I felt that energy taking me over now. My aunt continued talking as I went up the stairs to see my daughter for myself.

"Julie, she screamed. I mean a scream like I've never heard. So I ran up here as fast as I could. By the time I got up here, she was crying so hard that her face was red and her mouth was wide open but nothing was coming out." She went on still visibly upset.

"And so I picked her up and just held her, and finally she exhaled, but then, Julie, it got even weirder. She threw her body back in my arms, arching so much that I almost dropped her, and then I think she just passed out! She just went back to sleep, but it wasn't normal!"

I grabbed Emma gently from the crib where she appeared to be sleeping peacefully. She did not wake when I picked her up.

"Does she have another ear infection, Julie?"

"Good question," I replied calmly. It was likely the case. I thought perhaps her eardrum had burst again and checked carefully, but there was no evidence of that.

"You need to call 911 or take her to the emergency room right now! I was just on my way downstairs to call when you walked in the door. This just happened. Call her doctor now!"

I grabbed the phone and had her pediatrician paged, and within a few minutes I received a phone call. I hoped it was the same doctor who told me to pay better attention, but it wasn't. I was mad it wasn't him who had to call me back.

"It's probably just her ear again, Mrs. Obradovic," the doctor hypothesized. "Ear infections are very painful, especially at night when a child is lying down. There can be a lot of pressure, and with her history, I wouldn't be surprised if she's got a bad one again."

I told him that I wasn't there to hear it, but my aunt insisted this wasn't just a baby in a little bit of pain. She was certain something very serious had happened. I asked if we should go to the hospital.

"I really believe based on what you're telling me, and knowing her history, you're just dealing with more pain. If anything else happens, go straight to the emergency room, but if not, come in to the office first thing in the morning."

I told my aunt what he said, and she shook her head in disagreement. She begged me to go to the hospital and even offered to stay overnight if we wanted. I could tell she was upset and almost took her up on the offer, but the part of me that had become so used to doubting my own instincts took over. I decided to wait it out, and I assured my aunt that if anything else happened, we would go.

She was not happy with my decision. As she packed up her things, she pleaded, "Julie, I was a mother to two children and an aunt to all of you. I've watched tons of babies in my lifetime. I am telling you, in all of my life, I have never heard a child scream like that. Something is wrong."

And with that, she went home, and we went to bed. It was just past thirty days after Emma received her DTaP, pneumococcal, polio, and MMR vaccines while on another round of antibiotics.

It will all be over in a year

The next day, the doctors couldn't find evidence of anything unusual. Surprisingly, however, Emma did not have another ear infection. Whatever had caused her high-pitched screaming and arched back was not her ears, but no other explanation was offered or looked for.

Even so, the pediatrician thought it might be time to take a more drastic approach. He suggested we get ear tubes put in and explained it was a common and rather simple outpatient procedure. The tubes would allow her ears to drain if they filled with fluid, ideally preventing the fluid from getting infected. This was the hope.

I had heard of plenty of kids getting tubes by then, so I wasn't surprised at the suggestion. I actually welcomed it. The thought of no more antibiotics or frequent doctor visits was enticing.

We were given the name of an ear, nose, and throat specialist out of the affiliated hospital. A pediatric neurologist and developmental specialist were also in his office. The waiting room was full of children with problems. It scared me, and I thanked God for having a healthy child who only needed ear tubes.

The doctor walked us through the procedure and told us how to go about scheduling the surgery. He also asked if we had any questions. I had some, including why she had started putting her hands over her ears all the time now, but I kept them to myself. Questions and suggestions to doctors or nurses, I learned, were a no-no.

On December 16, 2002, Emma went under anesthetic to have tubes placed in both of her ears. In the surgical center, the staff went out of their way to make us comfortable. One nurse, who had given us gowns to wear as we waited in our room, took a Polaroid picture. I thought it was weird to document this event with a photo, but I was glad to have the picture later.

In it, Emma looks sad. She is wincing and has her hands over her ears, something she had started doing a lot lately. Later, the photo would prove to me something that I hadn't even noticed. Emma had stopped smiling.

Thankfully, the surgery went well. I was relieved and couldn't wait for the onslaught of infections to finally be over. I also couldn't wait for her to not be so sensitive to sound. She hated when I sang to her now, and she also hated the radio and the vacuum. I assumed her ear pain was the reason, and now that it would stop, so would her sensitivity.

All I wanted was for her to feel better, start talking better, and never be on antibiotics again. I wanted to put the whole nightmare behind us. I was so excited for that possibility.

Five days later, I gave Emma her bedtime bath. I was careful not to get any water in her ears and realized this was going to be a different difficulty to live with. I wrapped her in a bath towel, massaged her with the lotion recommended for her eczema, and brought her into her room to get ready for bed.

I then called Mike to get the camera. I remember being in a great mood, hopeful for our fresh start and eager to celebrate Christmas, which was only a few days away. I hadn't taken any pictures of her since Thanksgiving, and I wanted to be sure to capture the magic of every month.

He came in, sat in the glider chair, and started trying to get Emma to laugh for the camera. He couldn't. For at least a minute, he continued making funny faces and playing peek-a-boo. In the past, even when she was sick, that would always work. Now, there was nothing. She sat expressionless on the floor in front of him.

Finally, when I couldn't take it anymore, I decided to sit with her and try. I figured she just still didn't feel well and maybe needed Mommy to make her feel better. Frighteningly, my attempt didn't work either.

No matter what we did, no matter how many times we tried, Emma wouldn't smile or engage. And then I realized something. Not only hadn't she smiled since Mike's birthday, she hadn't spoken either. Until then, she didn't have a lot of words, but she had some. Now I couldn't remember the last time I heard her say one. We stopped taking pictures, and I quietly put her to bed.

That night, I knew my life had changed forever. The diagnosis and the devastation wouldn't officially come for almost another two years, but that was the night I knew. *I knew.* I knew beyond any doubt, beyond any doctor, beyond anything that anyone could tell me, something was wrong with my child.

My mom was right. My mother-in-law was right. My aunt was right. My grandmother was right. And I was right.

I lay on the side of my bed that faced her doorway and stared into the darkness of its direction. When I finally blinked, a tear rolled sideways down my cheek and into my ear as I talked myself out of my internal knowing to the best of my ability. I prayed as hard as I could, trying desperately to reassure myself everything was fine.

"It will all be over in a year," I kept repeating. "Everything will be okay in a year. Please, God, let everything be okay in a year."

That was the mantra I had adopted when life was so stressful five years earlier. But this time was different. I hoped it would be over in a year, that's for sure. But no matter how hard I tried to convince myself otherwise, I knew it wouldn't be. If anything, I knew her regression was just the beginning.

Chapter 3

Suspicion—A Moment of Weakness

In the fall of 2003, I got pregnant with our third child. I still wanted to have at least four and possibly five children. Now that Emma was experiencing so many health problems, however, I began to worry that might not be wise. At a minimum, I decided, I would have three. If she was seriously sick, she would need as much family as she could get.

Like my other pregnancies, this one was easy. I went into labor late at night, just like with Emma, and spent the evening waiting to give birth. When I got the epidural, which took nine times to get in, it slowed everything down. Not only was I forced to lie flat on my back because it wasn't working properly, I could still feel one half of my body.

At that point, though, I didn't really care. Allison was finally born in the morning, named after my godmother and her grandmother. She was out, and she was perfect, about the same size in weight and appearance as her brother had been.

Immediately, I looked over into the warming bed and waited for an instinct to hit me like it had with Emma. I worried tremendously that it would, but it did not. I knew right then she would be fine, the strongest of my three. I have never felt anything else since, and she has never been anything but.

Within a few hours, however, I could sense I was in for some trouble. My body was swelling. I couldn't put my slippers on because my feet were so fat. I never swelled after my first two children, and I was concerned.

I could also barely walk. My whole body hurt worse than with my first two births combined. I knew there was no way I was getting out of that hospital the next day like I had last time.

If anything, I was hoping to stay for a few days. Not only was I in worse shape, I had two other children to care for at home, one who was just about to switch from speech therapy in our home to speech therapy at the school. For the first time, I worried I had bitten off more than I could chew.

The Institute of Medicine

The day after Allison was born, I was watching television when a story confirming an Institute of Medicine ruling came on. The IOM had been asked by the Centers for Disease Control to independently review the scientific evidence linking either the vaccine preservative Thimerosal or the MMR vaccine to autism. Only three years earlier, in 2001, the IOM had concluded the theory was "biologically plausible." They were now reviewing science done in the interim to determine whether that was still the case.

I paid close attention because I had been loosely following the topic on some message boards I joined in an effort to see what was wrong with Emma. Just shy of her third birthday, someone suggested that Emma's adenoids were possibly swollen and that was why she was not only drooling so much but also having a hard time talking.

It seemed like a stretch, but I decided to investigate any connection. It was the most logical suggestion we had been given (someone had once sincerely advised it was likely her sippy-cup causing the problem).

Through my online search, I found a condition called apraxia. Apraxia is a speech motor disorder in which messages from the brain to the mouth are disrupted. Even though the muscles are fine, the person cannot move his or her lips or tongue properly to say sounds correctly. It can be caused by a stroke, traumatic brain injury, tumors, dementia, and other neurological disorders.

There were many similarities between the condition and what she was experiencing, including some co-morbid neurological signs, such as log-rolling. For the first time, I felt like we might be getting somewhere. I joined one of the online message boards dedicated to childhood apraxia to learn more.

Parents from around the world, mostly moms, shared their experiences, interventions, hypotheses, and more in an effort to help their children. They discussed supplements, diets, specialists, therapists, and therapeutic programs. It was the first place I felt hopeful there was something we could do; it was also where I finally felt my concerns were being taken seriously.

It was on this message board that someone mentioned vaccines playing a role in developmental disorders such as apraxia, and I remember being instantly annoyed by the comment. By then, I had completely forgotten about my earlier concern. It had been well over a year since Emma had had any vaccines, and besides, based on what I had read, it was a coincidence, that's all. Plus, I truly believed my doctors would have told me if it weren't. None of them had said a word.

And so I deleted those comments from the emails I would get daily on this board. Although I didn't pay close attention to that theory at that time, I was aware of it enough to have said something to my husband. I don't remember telling him anything specific, but I do remember this.

On the day we were going to be released from the hospital, I was asked to sign papers giving permission for Allison to receive a hepatitis B vaccine. Mike was in the room when they gave me the form and looked at me oddly.

"I thought we weren't going to give her that one?" he asked, concerned.

"No, it's fine," I replied confidently. "I just saw a report on television where they proved it."

On May 14, 2004, the Institute of Medicine made public the body of evidence suggesting Thimerosal, a mercury-based vaccine preservative, and the MMR, a triple live virus vaccine, had nothing to do with autism.

The IOM not only claimed it wasn't biologically plausible, a 180-degree turn from their position only three years earlier, they also said the evidence was so conclusive that no further research should ever be done on the subject. That was good enough for me. Our baby got her shot.

Red

A few days after I came home after giving birth to Allison, Emma began attending speech therapy through the school district. Once a child turns three years old, any developmental intervention they need that qualifies for services such as speech therapy becomes the responsibility of the school district they will eventually attend.

This is the law and something I knew nothing about until a fellow mother in the waiting room of the ear, nose, and throat specialist explained it to me. She also explained that the state offered Early Intervention Services in your home until the age of three if the child had certain developmental delays. All you had to do was call and make an appointment for an evaluation. She even gave me the number.

And so in the summer of 2003, still in the absence of any direction from our pediatricians, I made the call. Within a few weeks, several specialists came to our home to evaluate Emma across the board. When they finished, they informed me that she was significantly delayed in the areas of speech and language, appropriate play, and fine and gross motor skills. They did not, however, suggest autism as a concern.

Beginning immediately after their evaluation, a speech and developmental therapist from the state came to our home weekly to work with Emma. We also decided to hire a private speech therapist to do the same on a different day. For a minimum of two hours a week for over nine months, Emma got speech, language, and play-based therapy in our home. Regardless, it didn't help.

And so just before Allison was born, Emma had to be screened once again to see if she could now receive services from the school district. About a month before her third birthday in March 2004, I had to take her to the special education cooperative for another evaluation.

I sat on a bench in the hallway while they tested her speech and language, gross and fine motor skills, and social-emotional abilities. Emma still could not hold a conversation, play with a toy correctly, or show any evidence of imagination. She also remained uncoordinated and overly sensitive to sound, and she flapped her hands when excited. I knew she would qualify for services, equally grateful and heartbroken that she would.

To pass the time, I would look at the children's artwork displayed on the walls and think about projects I would implement when I went back to teaching that fall. I had taken that year off to have my third child.

Every once in a while, a class would march in front of me on their way to the gym. Most of the children were no more than eight years old. I would smile and wave as they giggled with one another, and then say a prayer. *Please, God, please let Emma have friends like that. Please let her be just like those little girls by that age. Please let everything be okay by then.*

After an hour, I was greeted by one of the teachers. She was kind, but she was concerned. She asked me if Emma zoned out often.

"Mrs. Obradovic, does Emma ever zone out and not respond to you? We were trying to do a few tests, and she just ignored us. I would wave my hand in front of her face, and there was nothing. It was like she was just gone, looking right through us. Are you aware of this?"

Yes, I was aware of it, as it was likely what my mother-in-law had described. There was also one time I put her in her car seat, and as I was buckling her, maybe a few inches from her face at most, I couldn't get her to look at me. I even said these words out loud, "Gosh, if I didn't know any better, I would swear you were autistic!"

But I never followed up on that suspicion. Of course, I didn't want her to have autism, but the fact that not a single doctor or therapist from one of the best hospitals in the country, or from the state's intervention specialists, or now from this school district, had suggested it, reassured me that I was wrong. And since I was always wrong, I kept my mouth shut.

The results of the testing weren't good. I didn't know exactly what they meant, but I knew enough to know they were suggesting brain damage. Emma showed evidence of low muscle tone. She was weaker on her right side, too. And they even asked me if she had ever had a stroke.

A stroke? Not that I knew of! But it was interesting they asked. The apraxia information I began researching mentioned it's a condition often seen in stroke patients. My curiosity was piqued. Could that have been what happened during her high-pitched screaming fit? I wondered.

They confirmed her significant speech delay. Although she could repeat and recite words, as she began saying words again about six months after the ear tube surgery, she could not put together any kind of pragmatic speech. There was no give and take, no abstract storytelling, no spontaneous speech, and no ability to properly answer many questions.

I also warned them not to ask her any predictable questions based on something I had just discovered. During one of the last in-home therapy sessions, the therapist showed me how well she was doing by asking basic questions like her name, her age, and her favorite color. She got all of them right.

Feeling suspicious later that day, however, I thought I would verify the progress. I worried that she had only learned the right response to a question, not the significance of what she was saying.

"Emma, how old are you?"

"Two."

"Yes, honey, that's right! Good job. And what's your favorite color?"

"Red."

"Oh, red! Yes, I like red, too! It's so pretty. Can I ask you another question? What's your favorite food?"

"Red."

"Red is your favorite food? Are you sure? What's your favorite toy?"

"Red!"

As I suspected, she had no idea what she was saying. She learned that the word "favorite" should be followed by the word "red." Since I was a foreign language teacher, her mistake was familiar to me.

When students are learning a second language, they will often choose a word or phrase based only on context, not meaning. In other words, they don't actually know what they are saying; they are just making a logical guess based on the context they recognize and a vague familiarity of having heard the word or expression used before.

This was exactly what Emma was doing—learning English as a foreign language. I immediately suspected the part of the brain that naturally learns a language at a young age wasn't working properly. When you are young, you don't have to think about this process. Your brain does it automatically. But as you grow older, that ability diminishes, and learning gets more difficult as we age. To me, this was the sign of a very serious concern.

I met with all of the teachers before we left. They discussed how the transition to the school district would take place and asked me to share any additional information they could use in developing her intervention plan. I shared that she just had a hearing test that proved no hearing loss. I also added that she was having her adenoids x-rayed to see if they were the reason that she was speech delayed and hyper-salivating.

I emphasized that I suspected apraxia and that one previous therapist thought it was, but another thought it was not. We had an appointment to see a third specialist to break the tie.

This therapist made a funny face, the kind of face you make when you think someone is way off base but don't really know what to say to correct her. She flat out rejected the notion Emma had apraxia, hinting that something else much more serious was going on.

When she didn't say what, however, I figured she didn't have any idea, just like everyone else. I did not know that neither she nor Early Intervention Services were allowed to suggest a diagnosis.

A weak episode

The first day of therapy through the school system, I dropped Emma off at the school where her speech-therapy sessions would take place now, no more than a half a mile from our home. It was the third week of May, and even though this was her first therapy session, it would likely be her last for the school year.

At home, my mom was helping me with the baby and the household. I was still in a tremendous amount of pain, unable to walk or sit comfortably even five days later. Although Allison was a wonderful little baby, I was overwhelmed, incredibly swollen, and exhausted. To add to it, my milk was coming in, and it hurt horribly. It was all I could do to get dressed to take Emma to the school.

Not ten minutes back in the house, the phone rang. A sweet southern drawl was on the other end, and I recognized it instantly. The same school nurse from when I had been a student was still working there. My heart began to race.

"Mrs. Obradovic," she began calmly. "Now, I don't want you to panic, okay, but we've had a little incident here, and I need you to come on up to the school immediately."

Emma wouldn't respond to her name or make eye contact, she claimed. In her professional opinion, she was having a seizure. She had called 911, and an ambulance would be there any moment. I needed to hurry.

A lump developed in my throat, and I could barely get the words out to tell my mother. She immediately calmed me down and made me focus, assuring me that she would be just fine with the baby; that she would make sure my son got home from school or even go get him if needed; that she would call Mike; and that right now, all I needed to do was get to the school as quickly as possible and call her when I knew what hospital we were going to.

On her orders, I waddled my swollen and achy body to the minivan and got to the school within minutes. Inside, they escorted me to the nurse's office, where Emma was lying on the bed. She looked no different from when I dropped her off, just scared and unsure of what was going on. I calmly approached, trying not to upset her.

The ambulance was already there by the time I arrived. A paramedic was talking to the nurse and the speech therapist, both retelling their version of events. Moments later, Emma was strapped to a gurney and wheeled outside. Junior-high students and staff members stared out the windows while we loaded up and left.

The sirens began blaring as we drove away, and poor Emma, who had not been upset in the slightest, was now getting anxious. She placed her hands over her ears and started to cry. I sang to her, forgetting she hated anyone singing, and tried my best not to cry, too, as I stroked her hair.

It's so hard to be strong when you are in such pain. Not only was I physically aching from having a baby, my heart was aching for Emma more and more with each passing day. Time, which I had always relied on, was making nothing better. It was actually only making things worse.

In the hospital, we were rushed to triage. Multiple doctors came from multiple places along with multiple nurses. It was so many people for such a small space, and they were working frantically in spite of the fact she was totally calm now. I worried they would make her upset again, and they did.

Not long after they began poking and prodding her, my husband arrived. I had no time to collapse in his arms before he was asked by the medical staff to help. Emma was so squirmy and worked up, they were going to have to strap her down to a body board. They figured if her daddy was there, she might be more cooperative.

She wasn't. It looked like she was being fixed to a crucifix, only a blue plastic one. I couldn't blame her for fighting them off. She wiggled her little body, thrashing about, screaming in fear, and completely uncooperative. There were at least three adults in addition to her father that had to hold her steady so she could be restrained. I nearly lost my mind watching them do it and was escorted out of the room by a nurse.

When the tests they needed were finally done, we had nothing to do but sit and wait. Following the blood draws and the urine sample via catheter, they now wanted to do some scans and an electroencephalogram (EEG). We would have to go to another part of the hospital, wait some more, do the tests, and wait some more. We were there for at least five or six hours.

Back in the room afterward, she was exhausted but in good spirits lying on the bed with Mike. She was calm now, resting comfortably with her daddy. He tried tickling her and distracting her to keep her entertained, and although she was tired, she was content.

I, however, on the other side of the room in a chair, was not faring as well. Now that the fear had mostly died down, and I also finally had the chance to sit down, my body was flooded with pain.

I felt achy, woozy, hot, and clammy. Instead of just my back, abdomen, and pelvis hurting, everything hurt.

My breasts were swelling, becoming hard and hot to the touch. There were also red patches developing on them. I needed my baby or a pump so badly, but there was no way to get either. For anyone to make the trip would be pointless. We would likely be home in an hour.

A nurse walked in to check on Emma and, catching a glimpse of me on her way out, asked if I was okay. I told her I was not, and that I had given birth only five days before. Her eyes widened as she whipped out a thermometer to take my temperature. I was burning up.

She scooted Emma and Mike off the bed and ordered me to lie down. She was going to go get a pump and a doctor immediately, fearing I had a breast infection. I gladly obliged and looked up into the bright fluorescent light.

I tried not thinking about what my little girl must have felt on that bed, strapped down, helpless, scared, and overwhelmed, but I couldn't help it. I finally let myself quietly and privately cry as I always did, the hot tears slowly making their way down the side of my cheeks to my ears once again. Everything, everything, everything hurt, most especially my heart.

One of the doctors returned shortly thereafter, but he was not there for me. He had the results of the tests, and he seemed disappointed. There was nothing abnormal. Emma's white blood cell count was a little high, but that was it. He called it a "weak episode" on the forms and sent us home, telling us to follow up with our pediatrician immediately.

We packed up our things, disgusted. All of this trauma, all of this testing, all of this time, and still nothing. Once again, nobody had any idea what was going on. It was getting beyond ridiculous, and I was frustrated and scared.

Meanwhile, the nurse who had taken my temperature came back in. She apologized but said she wouldn't be able to help me. Unless I was admitted as a patient, she wasn't allowed to do anything for me.

"Insurance," she said guiltily. "I'm so sorry."

She isn't getting better

As we were told, we immediately followed up with our pediatrician, who ordered a twenty-four-hour EEG. The neurologist was out of the same office as the ENT. We were now one of the families going to that office for other services.

That EEG was also negative for any seizure activity, just like the one in the hospital, which, although a good thing, actually made me feel worse. In spite of everything in her growing medical file that this new neurologist had access to, he offered no further suggestions about what could be wrong and ordered no further tests. It was as if because she had no seizure activity, there was nothing wrong, even though clearly something was.

I was desperate for answers by then, and becoming more convinced that no one had them. It's a frightening thing to have a sick child, that's for sure. It's an even more frightening thing to suspect no one knows how to help her. Worse, I would come to learn quickly enough, the repeated illnesses and infections, the loss of the ability to speak, the drooling, the low muscle tone and gait, and the eczema were only the beginning.

In spite of the fact we were seeing more doctors, getting more therapy, and having more testing, Emma was getting worse. That summer, she suffered two more ear infections, now a possible result of swimming in our pool. The tubes made her susceptible to swimmer's ear.

Worse than that, she was experiencing significant constipation. Her belly was substantially bloated, and her poops became hard and infrequent. One day, while I was just putting her in the tub, it started leaking out of her. We were told to try prune juice.

Not long afterwards, there was another poop episode, only this time it was in the pool. Thankfully, she had swimmer pants on, but even so, it created a terrible mess. My girlfriend, who had been in medical school and was now a doctor, told me I should get a prescription laxative. I thought it was odd no one seemed interested in getting to the cause of the problem but rather just offered me remedies for how to treat it.

And then that July, only two months after the previous hospital visit, we found ourselves back in the emergency room. One day, while Emma sat on the potty without going, I realized she looked sick. I took her temperature and confirmed she had a fever. Instantly, remembering the same symptoms in college, I knew that meant she had a urinary tract infection.

I grabbed her off the potty and raced to the hospital. Because she couldn't explain herself, I had no idea how long she had felt this way. I worried terribly that this had progressed to a dangerous point, and I felt awful that I had scolded her just before I realized what was going on. Although she had so many other problems, bathroom problems weren't really ever among them. Adding potty problems to our already big list just made me more afraid.

We got to the emergency room, and instead of being ushered into triage like last time, were ordered to the waiting room. Meanwhile, we were given a cup to get a sample. I looked at them like they had three heads. There was no way I was getting a sample. The girl couldn't pee.

I knew that meant they would have to catheterize her again, and I knew that meant they would have to hold her down. I was right on both counts, but I had not factored in that this time, I would be the one to hold her down. I did everything in my power not to cry or look her in the eyes while she screamed. My hope of not being a part of an episode of childhood trauma was being repeatedly dashed.

The results came back fairly quickly, and the doctor came in congratulating me. He complimented my intuition, which shocked me, and said he was surprised I figured out what she had. Sure enough, she had a kidney infection. There was even blood in her urine.

She was put on another powerful antibiotic, even though they lost the sample and never confirmed the bacteria that caused it. And at our follow-up with the pediatrician to check for kidney reflux, the test results came back negative. No one ever figured out why or how she got a kidney infection.

At home, I filled out the back cover of the baby book I had designated as the place to document my concerns about her health once again. By then, the list of illnesses, medications, reactions, and problems was long, as I originally suspected it would be. One whole side had been filled.

It had been almost three years since we started our journey down this road, I noticed as I reviewed it. In those three years since her first round of antibiotics at birth, she had been on at least twelve rounds of oral ones and several ear-drop kinds. Most had come within one year.

And the fact remained, staring back at me on the page, that no matter what we were doing—no matter how many tests, how many therapists, how many hospitals, how many doctors, or how many medications—one thing was very clear.

She wasn't getting better.

No, that's not normal

Over a year before the bladder infection, I asked my mom to come to the pediatrician with me for an appointment. Ever since the comment about paying better attention, I felt very uncomfortable, like I was a suspect, not Emma's mother. I knew I needed someone to speak up if I couldn't. That someone was my mom.

By the summer of 2003, she, like my mother-in-law, my grandmother, and my godmother, was convinced something was wrong. In February of that year, my mother had taken Emma to see a live performance of Disney's *Bear in the Big Blue House*.

According to my mom, Emma had a hard time paying attention. Instead, she stared at the ceiling fans. She also had to be taken out of the theater. She had been covering her ears the whole time, clearly uncomfortable and overwhelmed by the noise. My mom's description matched what I reported to the ear, nose, and throat specialist who assured me that her hearing was normal after we had it tested, and said that he had no idea why she might be covering her ears.

But there were other things, too. Because she also watched Emma for me while I worked, my mom saw the decline in Emma's development just like I did. She watched her go from a healthy, vibrant, babbling, bright-eyed, rosy-colored, strong baby to a somewhat weak, pale, distant-eyed, chronically sick child. She didn't like it any more than I did. And she made a very big deal out of Emma's repetitive shaking of her head.

I don't remember when it started, but Emma would be eating in her high chair, when all of a sudden, she would start shaking her head side-to-side, side-to-side. Sometimes she would even throw her arms behind her head and bang her head backwards. Sometimes she would do it while lying on the floor.

It didn't sit well with my mom, who wondered if she had a tic and insisted on going to the next appointment with me to validate my concerns. If these doctors didn't listen to me, maybe they would listen to her.

Alas, they did not. Mom was told the behavior was normal, but unlike me, who would simply keep my mouth shut, she was having none of it.

"I'm sorry, but no, that's not normal," she confronted the pediatrician confidently. "I have three children, umpteen nieces and nephews, that many more cousins of my own, and have been around children all my life. I've never seen a child do this. Ever."

It was the third woman of the three most important in my life to use the exact same words to explain their concern—my grandmother, my godmother, and now my mother. He said something in reply to dismiss her, and that was the end of it. We packed our things, and she paused to address me as we walked out of the room.

"You need new doctors, Julie."

I knew my mom was probably right, but the thought of getting new doctors seemed like a crazy idea. Emma's medical file was huge, and whether I liked them or not, her current ones had known her since birth.

I was insulted by the one comment to pay better attention to my daughter, yes, but I didn't think they were bad people. In fact, the new pediatrician they just welcomed to the group was wonderful. I liked him a lot. And they practiced out of one of the best hospitals in the country. The idea that anyone else would know something they didn't seemed unlikely.

So I stayed with them. But after the twenty-four-hour EEG the following summer, the second one to show that nothing was abnormal, I thought it might be time to get a second opinion. One day, while listening to an annual radio telethon for another hospital, I decided to make a call. Perhaps a hospital that specialized only in children's health would hold more answers, I reasoned.

Yes, my doctors were affiliated with an incredible medical institution. And yes, it was probably a waste of my time. But just in case, I figured, I would see what another neurologist had to say.

I picked up the phone and dialed the number on the website. After going through several steps with several people, I was given an appointment. The soonest we could see someone was February—more than four months away.

Institute Day

It was the day after parent-teacher conferences at the end of the first quarter, and we were stuck in meetings all day. I had finally gotten back to work that fall after taking a leave the year before to have Allison. It was the first school year I began to experience a love-hate relationship with my career that would last until I left education twelve years later.

Initially, I was very happy to be back. I was exceptional at what I did, and without conceit, I knew it. I could feel it. In the classroom,

I was always my most authentic self. And I had big plans for my career. I had just completed my first master's degree the prior year. I intended to get at least one more master's in administration and, after that, a doctorate, preferably from Harvard. I wanted to be the best Spanish teacher on the planet, and I intended to be so, as well as a graduate professor of education.

To add to my enthusiasm, teaching was a form of respite from the demands on me at home. I had to be fully present while teaching, which made it impossible to think about other things . . . like a sick child no one seemed to know anything about.

But that year, ironically, for the first time and for the very same reasons, I began to struggle with my career choices. *Teaching made it impossible to think about other things . . . like a sick child no one seemed to know anything about.* I felt guilty now that my time was not fully dedicated to Emma, taking care of her and figuring out what was wrong. I felt guilty that I had to rely on my mother and mother-in-law to get her on and off the little bus to her Early Intervention preschool program.

I had wrestled a little with working-mom guilt from the time my son was born, but this was different. Working away from home when you have healthy, normally developing children is one thing. Working away from home when you don't is quite another. To me, it felt significantly worse.

On this day, however, it was still too soon to know how much of a toll trying to maintain my career while meeting Emma's needs would eventually take on me. Guilt like this was still fresh, and not a feeling I knew intimately.

To cope, I made a conscious decision to ignore my guilt while teaching and concentrate on being the best teacher I could instead. At school, I reasoned, I needed to focus on school. At home, I needed to focus on home. Naively, I thought it was that simple.

In between Institute Day professional development sessions, I went to the faculty lounge to check my messages. Our school did not have phones in any of the teachers' rooms, so if you wanted to check your voicemail, you had to make a special trip.

It was annoying and stressful. The lounge was not close to my room, so I didn't always go there. There would admittedly be days I would forget to check my messages, and there would be nothing worse than coming in worried that I had missed a parent's call.

And so this Friday at the end of October 2004, I made sure to check if anyone had called. Although parent-teacher conferences were held the day before, it was possible a parent who hadn't been able to make it needed to speak to me.

Sure enough, as I feared, there was a message. My heart raced as I pressed the button to listen to it. You just never know what's going to be on the other side of that call, and this was certainly one of those times.

"Hi, Julie, this is Sally Lou Loveman from *The Oprah Winfrey Show*," said a kind and joyful voice from the end of the receiver. I pulled it away from my ear and looked at it in disbelief.

"I was calling to let you know that Oprah read your letter and loved it! She would like to invite you to be on an upcoming show. Please call me as soon as possible so we can discuss the details."

I stood there in shock, my heart racing even faster now. *Oprah? What letter?* I thought for a second, confused. Oh, *that* letter, I remembered. *That letter*?

Without giving it too much more thought, I frantically called her back. Sure enough, Oprah had invited me to be on her program. She had read my letter and wanted to invite me to a show she was doing for teachers. We went over the rest of the details, which were numerous, and I hung up the phone in shock.

I stood there for a moment, not sure how to tell anyone what had just happened, when something even more amazing dawned on me.

The date of the taping was Saturday, November 20. I knew exactly what show this was going to be. I reached for the sofa behind me and carefully sat down.

I was the one having a weak episode now.

Chapter 4

Confirmation—Sometimes When We're Disappointed . . .

Four times a year, I have to buy my mother a present: Mother's Day, anniversary, birthday, and Christmas, in that order. And four times a year, I have no idea what to get her. It gets harder every time.

In the summer of 2004, just before her birthday, she had an idea. She would love tickets to *The Oprah Winfrey Show*. That afternoon I got right to work. After a few minutes, however, I realized it wasn't going to be possible. You couldn't just buy tickets.

Defeated, I stayed on the web page a little longer, looking at articles and checking out the upcoming shows. That's when I saw it, a little box on the side of the home page asking if I was a teacher. I clicked on it and started responding to questions.

What was my best teaching moment? What was my worst? What did I believe my role was in children's lives? It felt like an application, not a survey, and the more time I spent on it, the more I felt obligated to finish. Even so, I was somewhat annoyed. I had not been prepared to write several lengthy and personal essays.

After I finished, I reread what I wrote, feeling proud. I loved my career and was grateful I had a profession that was meaningful. I was also proud of the work I was doing. My worst moment was finding a young woman in the bathroom contemplating suicide. I submitted the letter and never thought about it again until the day I got the call.

Within moments of speaking with the producer, I became giddy. I knew exactly what show this was going to be: "Oprah's Favorite Things." I had been home on leave the year before, and I watched the show religiously. By 2003, everyone knew being on her "Favorite Things" show was like winning the lottery.

Coincidentally, the day that show aired, I made a promise to myself. Somehow, someway, I was going to get on it. All I had to do was figure out when they did the taping, I assumed, and just make sure to get tickets for that time of year. I made a mental note that it was November.

I sat on the sofa speechless. Not only was this taping in November, but it was also for teachers. Oprah loved teachers. Even better, she had just given away those cars the month before. She was in a very philanthropic place, and now, I imagined, she wanted to target specific audiences with her generosity. She was giving her "Favorite Things" to teachers. I knew it with every fiber of my being.

But as excited as I was, there was a problem. I could only bring a working, certified teacher as my guest. My mother, a former dental hygienist and current paralegal, wouldn't be able to go. I decided to invite my cousin, an elementary school teacher, instead.

The show taped on a Saturday morning. Oprah likely didn't want to be accused of taking several hundred teachers out of their classrooms and costing school districts thousands of dollars in substitute pay. I couldn't blame her.

And so the Friday before, still thoroughly convinced I was going to be a part of the "Favorite Things" show, I was gathering my things for school when a commercial for *The Oprah Winfrey Show* aired. On the screen an audience was being showered with gifts. The "Favorite Things" show was going to air Monday.

I dropped my bag and stood for a moment completely crushed. That was not last year's audience. And the show airing Monday was already taped. I had been wrong.

I felt sorry for myself for a few minutes, but not much more. I reminded myself that I was lucky to be going to the show anyway, and that really, this wasn't about getting presents. I even felt guilty for getting so focused on that.

"Oh well," I thought as I went to work that day. I still get to meet Oprah! And she liked my letter.

Early the next morning, we headed to Harpo Studios. We were anxious when they finally let us enter to choose our seats, and we went for the center back row in order to be able to see everything. As I looked around, I glanced at the ceiling. Suspended above us were trees, ornaments, and all kinds of holiday decorations.

"Look," I nudged my cousin. "I was right. They already taped it."

There's this boy in my class . . .

In many ways, I am so happy I was unprepared for what happened next. That I was completely positive it was the "Favorite Things" show, followed by the let-down of being completely positive it wasn't, and then completely surprised by the fact that, after all, yes, it was . . . well, that was the experience of a lifetime. I now know it was also the gift of a lifetime.

When Oprah stated that because teachers give so much to their students, she wanted to give us "the hottest ticket in television," I thought I would lose my mind. The entire audience began screaming and jumping up and down, literally losing their minds. It was complete pandemonium. We lost our voices and our breath in a matter of minutes. I have never experienced anything like it.

We called everyone in our family immediately afterward on the way home, going over in detail the thousands of dollars of gifts we had received: a laptop, a navigation system, a flat-screen television, a trip to a spa, and so much more. We actually had a headache from the joy, and our faces hurt from smiling.

By the time we finished calling everyone, we were almost home. Not having anything else to add, my cousin changed the topic. She asked how Emma was doing.

I wasn't surprised by her question. The whole family knew by then that something bad was happening, and I suspected that many of my family members thought I was in denial, assumed I had stupid doctors, knew something I didn't, or all three. As an elementary school teacher, my cousin was concerned.

"You know, there's this boy in my class," she started softly. "Emma reminds me a lot of him."

I took the bait and a deep breath.

"Well, he's got sound sensitivity, and he needs to wear headphones to block it out sometimes. And he's got a pretty bad speech delay, flaps his hands, and a lot of other stuff really similar to her. Only he has a diagnosis of PDD."

"PDD? What's that?" I had never heard of it before and became extremely excited at the possibility of being pointed in the right direction.

"It stands for pervasive developmental disorder. It's basically another word for autism, but there are several different kinds. I think you'd be wise to look into it."

I didn't need to look into it. I knew right in that moment I had my answer. The answer I hoped for, prayed for, and dismissed for almost two years. The answer I knew in my heart from the day I put her in the car seat and she wouldn't make eye contact. The answer I knew the night she wouldn't smile for the camera. The answer I kept waiting for one of the doctors to give me, but never got.

I stared out the window in silence the rest of the car ride home. Oprah and everything that had just happened, all of the joy, all of the excitement, all of it was gone. It was replaced by the familiar feelings of anxiety, fear, and panic that I carried with me almost every moment of every day now.

Watching the cars pass by, I realized what had just happened. I looked to the heavens and shook my head in understanding. I knew how impossible it was to have just gotten on *The Oprah Winfrey Show*. I knew how incredible it was, what I had just experienced.

It wasn't a coincidence. It wasn't an accident. God gave me something wonderful to remind me that life still had joy. He wanted me to have something great before my world turned upside down. This I knew for sure.

I emptied the bags from her trunk and came in the house. I placed them right on the floor and walked over to the computer to do a Google search. Thankfully, my husband and kids were not home.

"P-D-D."

Within seconds, there were pages of information about it. I looked for one that showed the actual diagnostic, clinical criteria from the *Diagnostic and Statistical Manual of Mental Disorders, Fourth Edition*, and clicked on it. In front of me was a perfect description of everything wrong with my daughter.

I stared at it in horror. In less than a few hours, I had experienced one of the greatest moments of my life, and now, my very worst. Emma had autism.

I'll cry about this later

There were no tears, no screams, and no sounds that came out of me in that moment. I was completely paralyzed. For several minutes, I just stared at the description of the disorder with my hands folded together pressed up against my lips. I couldn't tell if I felt relieved, afraid, confused, or all three. Whatever the answer, it was quickly replaced by something else.

"How did everyone miss this?" I banged my fist on the desk in front of me. "How the fuck did everyone miss this?"

I got up and slammed the office chair into its space. Standing now, I paced around in small circles bitching out loud to no one like I always do when I'm angry.

"How many specialists have we been to? How many therapists? How many tests have we done? How many damn times have I told these people something was wrong?"

The list of questions I had for the universe seemed endless. I couldn't understand how this much time had passed with no answers. All these years, all this suffering, all these specialists, and all it took was a stupid Google search!

And once again, I had been right. I had been right! Not the doctors. Not the therapists. I had known! They didn't know their head from a hole in the ground, I lamented.

The anger subsided momentarily, and I abruptly felt fear and sadness enveloping me. The magnitude of what this meant was washing over me, and just like in the hospital, I felt woozy, hot, and clammy. I thought I would pass out. I grabbed the office chair and sat on it, folded in half with my head between my knees for about five seconds.

I then sat straight up. Like the night Emma had the high-pitched screaming fit, I became eerily calm, which meant only one thing. This was life or death. There was no room for any other emotion than resolve. I had to think, and I had to think fast. When the house is on fire, you don't sit around and cry about it. You get the hell out.

I scooted in the office chair and went back to the computer. As I stared at the screen once again, I said these last words aloud.

"I will cry about this later. Right now, there's work to do."

It would be six years before later finally came.

Giving thanks

From that moment forward, I really didn't care about being on *The Oprah Winfrey Show*. It seemed so unimportant. I sent an email to my closest friends and family telling them to watch it, but nothing more. Even at school, I didn't say a word except to a few people. Most were surprised at how uninterested in advertising my experience I seemed.

In hindsight, I may have come across like an ungrateful brat. I really don't know. All I do know is that I was in a haze. It felt like I was in the twilight zone, kind of like watching myself from the outside. I now believe I was in shock.

To add to it, that week was Thanksgiving. Mike and I had agreed to host the event and were expecting a large crowd. I had to teach, shop, clean, prepare, and cook all while taking care of three small children, one of whom I had just learned very likely had autism.

It was the last thing I wanted to do, and the idea of having to discuss this new information with anyone seemed torturous. I would have to put on a good show, I decided, but unfortunately, I wasn't that good of an actress.

Two years earlier, I was the one who said the Thanksgiving prayer before the meal. Around that time, I came up with a simple one based on a church marquee that suggested trying to pray without asking for anything.

The only way you could really do that was to say what you were grateful for instead. And so I made up a little prayer that I had been saying nightly since. I said it at Thanksgiving that year.

> *Dear God,*
> *Thank you for keeping us safe, happy, healthy, and free from suffering. Please continue to do so in the coming year.*
> *Amen.*

Truth be told, I hoped that by believing we were safe, happy, healthy, and free from suffering we actually would be fine forever. But as Emma slipped further away, and as her health became more complex, I felt like I was trying to trick God. Like I could will her health into existence by pretending it was already there. Obviously, I realized, you can't trick God.

Thanksgiving night at our house, I couldn't say the prayer. We weren't safe. We weren't happy. We weren't healthy. And we certainly weren't free from suffering. I asked Mike to say grace instead and escaped to my room for some privacy and a chance to breathe. I stayed in my bathroom for several minutes just trying to focus.

When I walked back into my room, my aunt was there (the one who had been babysitting when the high-pitched scream occurred; she was also the mother of my cousin who had gone to *Oprah* with me). She was looking for her coat among the ones piled on my bed.

"Hey, how are you doing?" she asked slowly and sincerely. I could tell from the way she tilted her head when she asked that she knew what was going on.

"I'm fine," I lied in my most pretend-upbeat voice while trying not to look at her, helping her find her coat. "I mean, I'm a little tired from all of this, but I'm okay."

She looked at me and moved so she was standing squarely in front of me.

"I talked to your cousin. I know what she told you."

I had nothing to say in response.

"So, I'm going to ask you again, how are you doing?"

"I'm okay," I barely got out the words before a massive lump filled my throat and the tears started welling in my eyes. She came close and wrapped her arms around me, but I let her hold me only for a second. I could feel my body going weak and knew if I let my pain come up, I would fall apart. I would not let that happen. I took a deep breath and a step backward out of her embrace.

"It's okay to be overwhelmed, Julie. This is a lot to take. We're all here for you. You know that, right?"

"I know. And thank you, I appreciate that. But really, I'm okay," I lied again, rummaging through the coats.

"We've got a lot of work to do," I continued again in my upbeat voice. "In fact, I already have a few appointments scheduled. I want to get moving on this as quickly as possible."

"Well, would it be okay if I went to an appointment with you? I'd like to be a part of this, if you'll let me."

"That would be great. It really would."

I found her coat, put on a smile, and said I had to get back downstairs to the party. I still remember her standing there, shaking her head at me, another person appearing to know something I didn't.

"Oh, honey. I'm worried about you."

"Don't worry about me," I begged as I headed down the stairs. "I'm fine. Worry about Emma."

The not-so-most wonderful time of year

Christmas arrived within weeks. My mind was a blur processing what I had confirmed about Emma, trying to figure out what to do about it, researching how it may have happened, finishing out the semester teaching, managing the lives of three children under the age of six, getting one back and forth to preschool and therapy, running a household, trying to be a good wife, and attempting to create a joyous Christmas for us all.

It was nearly impossible. Christmas had always been my favorite time of year, but this year, I dreaded it. My almost four-year-old daughter could barely speak, which meant she couldn't tell me what she wanted. By four, her brother had a list a mile long and a healthy interest in Thomas the Tank Engine. He knew the names of the engines and numbers by heart.

Emma had no such interests. If anything, she had no ability to use her imagination. She didn't play with toys properly, if at all. She twirled things, spun them, and turned them upside down. She liked to watch fans spin and play with light switches and doorknobs.

She could be destructive, and she had no idea how to share. She barely even noticed other people in the room with her. And she certainly couldn't name anything she liked. I still had no idea what her favorite color was, having confirmed "red" was a rote response.

These were the little things, among so many more that autism would eventually present, that would be among the hardest to handle. The normal milestones of a child, their first words, their favorite movies and characters, and their favorite toys, you would never know.

What they wanted for their birthday, what cake flavor they liked or didn't like, and the cute or funny mispronunciations or quirks they would have as a toddler, you would never know. Their personality, their silly nature, and their sense of humor, you would never know. The sound of their voice in a conversation with you, you would never know.

The sense of loss and heartbreak was indescribable, mothering this beautiful child locked inside. I couldn't imagine carrying this pain for the rest of my life, but I couldn't imagine I ever wouldn't. In fact, I worried it would only get worse.

I began noticing healthy three-year-olds everywhere, bombarded by the differences. It got so bad that I often didn't want to be in any place where I would see children the same age as Emma. Many times, I still don't. It was the beginning of an assault on my soul that has not ended to this day.

All I know is . . .

We headed out on Christmas Eve early as we always had. First, we went to my husband's family, then church, and then my family. To begin the stressful day, a conversation with a relative went south. I cautiously began confiding what I was learning about Emma and what we believed was wrong. I was nervous to say the words aloud, let alone to discuss it with anyone.

It was then she told me she had known that my daughter had autism for years. Just like that, matter of fact, she claimed to have known what we didn't, what Emma's doctors didn't, and what I had actually also suspected for just as long.

I lost my breath as she said it, trying to determine if I was more pissed off at the nerve and insensitivity it took to say this to my face, or the idea that maybe she really did know all this time and didn't say anything. Neither possibility made me feel better. I smiled and asked Mike if we could leave shortly thereafter.

After church, we went to my grandmother's. We were all quite tired by the time we arrived, and I was emotionally wrecked. I just wanted to leave, to be alone in a small room and turn out the lights. It was the first time I craved to be alone in the dark.

To keep safe, I isolated myself with Emma to the front hall closet, where my grandmother kept the few toys she had. If I could just avoid my family, I hoped, I might not say something I'd regret. It didn't work.

My mother came over to sit with us and then my cousin and then my grandmother. Emma sat in the middle, taking the toy in front of her and examining it, not playing with it, as usual. She spun it around, picked it up and dropped it, then slammed it on the floor with a thud. My heart broke into more pieces with it.

"Why does she do that, Julie?" asked my mother, concerned. "What are the doctors telling you? Why doesn't she play with her toys normally?"

My grandmother, who had watched Emma for two years once a week while I got my first master's degree, echoed her sentiment.

It was a legitimate question coming from a good place. My mom was not only watching Emma suffer without help, she was watching me. She, too, was frustrated. I hadn't considered how hard it is for grandparents to deal with autism, watching their children and grandchildren struggle, and wouldn't for many years to come. So I lashed out in anger.

"I don't know!" I growled through gritted teeth. I could feel the rage in my eyes and my heart, and I could feel that it was misplaced. I didn't care.

"I don't know why she does what she does, okay? And in spite of what everyone else seems to think, neither do any of you!"

She looked at me, wide-eyed and confused, clearly unable to figure out where any of this was coming from. I offered no explanation and looked at my grandmother.

"I don't know why she's doing anything that she's doing!" I was yelling by this point, my voice quaking more with each word, the lump in my throat too big to hold back the tears much longer.

"I don't know why any of this is happening," I held on to my voice by lowering it and my eyes. By the next sentence, I could no longer do so.

"All I know is . . ." I began to sob.

"All I know is this whole thing started with an ear infection . . ." I grabbed Emma and held her to me tightly, ". . . and now . . . it's autism."

My mom grabbed us both and let me cry in her arms.

Sometimes, when we're disappointed . . .

By February, my whole world had changed. I learned an enormous amount about autism, and how I might be able to help Emma. I spent the majority of my time on the computer, the house going to hell, the kids and my husband feeling neglected, and my thoughts occupied exclusively by autism.

I felt panicked but hopeful, anxious to get the official diagnosis, and I assumed it was a neurologist who made that call, which is why I wanted a second opinion. At no point yet had I been referred to a developmental pediatrician. Finding out later that one shared an office with our ear, nose, and throat doctor and first neurologist, both of whom very easily could have just walked us down the hall, incensed me.

My appointment with the second neurologist finally arrived, the one I made back in the fall. Whereas I had originally intended it to point me in the right direction, I now intended it to give me the right diagnosis.

To help, I crafted a several-page document of her medical history with dates, vaccinations, medications, and symptoms as they appeared in chronological order. I also brought a copy of the clinical criteria for PDD. I really just needed this doctor to confirm my suspicion. With my information, I couldn't imagine he wouldn't.

I waited with my youngest as she slept in her car seat in the private examining room while Emma was assessed. She was asked to walk up and down the hallway several times. She also had to perform a number of additional tasks. The doctor, an older man, came back into the room with a smile when they were done.

I came at him with a number of questions. I had waited months for this appointment, and I wanted them answered immediately. Unfortunately, I would have to wait some more. In spite of the fact I had provided him with a detailed medical history, he wanted me to dictate it to him instead. It seemed insane, and I grew irritated.

As I read word for word from the existing document, Emma sat on a stool in the corner *stimming*—the name for any repetitive, self-soothing behavior. Emma particularly loved to rock back and forth incessantly when sitting. She was actually somewhat obsessed with rocking, I felt. In fact, she would only sleep in our rocking chair at home, and she still tried to crawl into her baby swing that Allison was now using. I pointed out the rocking to the doctor, but he didn't seem to think it mattered.

An alarm arose in my belly. This appointment wasn't going to be what I had expected. I continued reading to him anyway, when he turned on his stool and made a T with his hands.

"Time out, mom," he said with a smile. "You're going too fast, and a lot of this is unnecessary."

Time out? What am I, five? And don't call me mom, asshole.

My belly burned hotter, my patience for anyone almost nonexistent. Son of a bitch, it was happening again.

"Exactly what part of this information is unnecessary?" I didn't let him answer and started listing many of her symptoms on the page in front of me.

"This child has been repeatedly and chronically ill for years, has been hospitalized for suspected seizures, has terrible eczema on her arms and legs, has dark circles under her eyes all the time, can't talk in complete sentences or hold any kind of conversation, has no evidence of imaginary play, doesn't know how to play with a toy properly, is completely uninterested in her peers, or anyone for that matter, loves to rock nonstop and sleep in a rocking chair, can't stand the sound of a vacuum or singing, flaps her arms like a bird when she's excited, is fascinated by fans and door knobs, has haphazard eye contact at best, and is sitting on that stool over there stimming to self-soothe. What part of that are you uninterested in?"

"Mom, mom, mom," he said again, trying to reassure me he meant no harm and no offense. "I don't mean any of that is unimportant. I just mean all of the dates and details are not. I get the big picture."

"Okay, sorry," I apologized, feeling stupid and rude. I remembered that I desperately needed his help and tried again to be nice.

"So if you get the big picture, what do you think is going on? Am I right? Is it PDD? Is it autism?" He turned back around to write something in her file.

"It certainly seems like it, yes, but trust me, you don't want it to be PDD," he replied without looking at me.

Well, no shit, Sherlock. No one wants it to be cancer, either. That doesn't mean it isn't.

"What does that mean?"

"Well, you know, mom . . ." he rolled his stool close to me as if to comfort me. "Sometimes when we are disappointed in our children, they can manifest that disappointment as a delay."

I looked at him dumbfounded. Was he suggesting my daughter was presenting with all of the things I told him because I was *disappointed* in her? No, it couldn't be, I decided, certain I must have misunderstood him.

"Here," he handed me a business card. "This is the name of a therapist I think you and your husband would benefit from seeing."

I hadn't misunderstood anything. He was suggesting our disappointment was at the root of Emma's problems. It was the craziest thing I had ever heard, and I made the face of someone with that thought as I took the card. Any politeness still in me had left the room.

"Wait, wait . . ." I said, half laughing, half stunned. "You think Emma is the way she is because my husband and I are disappointed in her?"

"No, no, not exactly. What I mean is that she may start to pick up on the disappointment you have in her developmental delays, and that may perpetuate them." It was pretty much the exact same sentence.

"But I can't say for sure. This psychologist can. That's why I think you should see her. The whole family would benefit, truly."

I held the card in my hand and stared at it blankly while he babbled on about getting a summary written and submitted to our pediatricians. He offered no guidance on how to move forward, no explanation for why a psychologist could be the one to help diagnose autism (if that's even why he referred us to one), no insight about the suspected seizures, and no suggestions about the inability to speak pragmatically. Instead he just told me how to go about checking out and wished us well. I put on my coat, grabbed the diaper bag, and helped Emma off the stool where she was still stimming.

In the minivan, I sat on my hands and waited for the heat to kick in while I contemplated what had just happened. Staring at my daughters through the rearview mirror, I confirmed things were even worse than I thought.

Emma had autism or something like it. No one at some of the best hospitals in the country appeared to know how to diagnose her or help her. And for whatever crazy reason I had yet to understand, this doctor was blaming me.

PART II

THE DECISIONS

Chapter 5

Panic—Getting Away

I lay awake uncomfortable in the queen-size bed for most of the night. To my right, Emma lay sprawled out in her footie pajamas. She took up most of the bed, but I didn't care. The fact she was sleeping at all was wonderful. There was no rocking chair in this hotel room, the only place she would sleep at home.

To my left, in the small space between the second queen-size bed where my husband and our son slept, was our playpen. Our youngest daughter, not yet a year old, spent the evening there. She too was fast asleep.

I, however, could not sleep. After having children, I became an incredibly light sleeper. Coupled with the anxiety of what was happening to Emma—I was always keeping one ear open for her—it made sleep a rare commodity for me.

Right on schedule, the baby began to stir. She wiggled her way off of her sheet, her pajamas making a swooshing sound on the play mat as she moved. I hoped that if I lay perfectly still and did not catch her eye, she would go back to sleep. I was not yet ready to face another day at the massive indoor water park where we stayed.

My hopes were quickly dashed. Allison was ready to get up and whimpered just enough to wake Mike. He gently lifted her out of the playpen, brought her to the dressing area with him, and returned within a minute wearing jeans and a ball cap.

Without saying a word, he grabbed the double stroller, placed our daughter inside, and left the room. I had no idea where they were going, but I was grateful they had left. I instantly felt my body relax.

Within a few minutes I dozed off deeply. I knew I didn't have long to enjoy the rest, but I savored the peace and relaxation that had taken over my mind and body with one less child to worry about. It was why I didn't register the soft click in the background for several minutes until after I heard it.

Click.

Just like that. Someone had opened the door and closed it gently behind them. Mike, I assumed for a moment, but then remembered it couldn't have been. He was gone. Housekeeping, I assumed second, and then realized it was way too early. Suddenly, in a flash, I knew.

I bolted straight up, the most massive adrenaline shot I have ever felt pulsing through my body. To my left, I could make out the shape of a little boy wrapped in blankets sleeping quietly. My son was safe.

To my right, however, there was nothing. Although I could see the empty space beside me, I slapped my hand up and down the area to feel for a body anyway, hoping she scooted down to the bottom. I then dove across her side of the bed to see if she had fallen on the floor. No luck. Emma was gone.

I sprang to my feet from the other side of the bed where I hung over looking at the floor. I stood for a moment, slightly crouched, legs apart, arms and hands out to the sides, looking left and then right and then left and then right like someone who needed to escape.

I needed to get out of the room as quickly as possible, but suitcases, toys, towels, clothes, floaters, and the cooler we brought with us created an obstacle course. I made my way past them clumsily and bolted for the door. A few steps away, I realized I couldn't see.

Glasses! My glasses! Where the hell are my glasses?

I went back to the minefield and fumbled loudly through our things on the desk to no avail, deciding I would have to go without them. Every second was a second she was alone. I had my hand on the door when another thought stopped me cold.

My son! What am I going to do with him?

Rousing him and bringing him with me would take too long, but leaving him alone, to possibly wake without anyone in the room, could be terrifying. I had to hope he would stay asleep. I swiped the room key from the desk to make sure I could lock him in and left. Stepping into the hallway, I faced yet another decision.

Which way would she go?

We were in one of the largest indoor water parks in the world. Determined to put autism out of our minds and spend some quality family time together, we had taken a four-hour drive north to get away. I had never seen a place as massive as this, buildings of hotel rooms with three to four floors each, all connected to restaurants, golf courses, lakes, walkways, arcades, shops, and enormous outdoor and indoor pools.

In a matter of minutes, almost four-year-old Emma could be anywhere. We were on the first floor of the main building. If she went right, a short walk down the hall would lead her outside to the parking lot. If she went left, a long walk down the hall would lead her to the elevators, stairs, an arcade, and one of the many pools.

My instinct told me she would go left, and I took off in that direction. Until that moment it hadn't dawned on me this would be the last place we could escape the dangers autism presented.

The hallway remains for me a vision of what a nightmare feels like. It was blurry (without my glasses) and dimly lit. For hundreds of yards, there were no windows. Since the hotel catered to families, the carpet was brightly colored and themed, the pattern repeating beneath my feet every few steps, all of it swirling together.

It seemed to go on forever, the same doors on either side of me passing by over and over and over again. In spite of being out of breath while I sprinted, I called Emma's name as loudly as I could.

"Emma! Emmie!" I yelled as I made my way toward the pool. I worried momentarily that I would wake the other people on the floor, but I didn't care anymore. She had to hear me before she could see me. I continued calling her name, trying to hold back tears.

Suddenly, still quite far away, I could make out a change in the hallway. Something like a stairway was off to the right, some vending machines beside it, and off center to the left of both, a sitting area with arcade games surrounded by windows to an indoor pool.

As I approached, I encountered other people for the first time. The stairway led up to the coffee bar on the second floor. Families were making their way up and down with their drinks. I must have looked like a mad woman as I entered their space at lightning speed, crying, squinting, and in my pajamas.

A man on a sofa saw me coming. With a calmness that irritated me, he pointed at me and then at something else. As I got closer, I saw he was sipping coffee with a stroller in front of him. I wondered if he was giving me the finger when I realized it was Mike.

"Mike!" I shouted breathless. "Emma's gone! She left the room while I was sleeping! We have to find her!"

By now I was in full panic mode, and I could no longer hold back the tears. Without saying a word, he simply made the same gesture, lifting his arm and pointing to something behind him. I could not yet figure out why he wasn't panicking.

And then I saw her. Emma, still in her footie pajamas, sat happily on the racecar machine waiting for it to give her a ride. Mike had given her a quarter, and even though the ride was over, she wouldn't get off. I ran to her, grabbed her, and fell to my knees with her in my arms.

"Emma, don't ever do that again!" I scolded with relief, love, and fear. "Don't ever leave without telling Mommy, do you understand?"

In that moment, I had no idea if she understood or not, but I did. I understood that my daughter was at risk for getting away from us quite easily. I understood that as a barely verbal, non-conversational child, she was in even more danger than a young child already is. And I understood that my perception of what we would be able to enjoy and do as a family had changed forever.

I brought her to Mike where he shared that he had gotten coffee upstairs with the baby, and that precisely when the elevator door opened on his return to our floor, he happened to see her walk right by. She was headed to the pool.

I stood for a moment, stunned at the extraordinary chance of that happening, when I remembered our son was still alone in our room asleep. After securing Emma with Mike, I took off sprinting back down the hallway and entered to find him exactly as he was when I left. I had been gone for less than five minutes.

Chapter 6

Investigation—There's a Book?

As I began to research how to help Emma, an episode from my son's infancy replayed in my head. Although he was initially a very happy baby, something had gone terribly wrong by the end of his first month. It was colic, more than one person told me, a mysterious yet common affliction that for some unknown reason made babies gassy and miserable.

My mother insisted we get out into the world anyway and picked us up on a weekday to head to a local shopping mall. We tried to enjoy ourselves while strolling, but my son was having no part of it. Eventually, we needed to find some privacy.

We found it in a very fancy women's room with a lovely sitting area where I checked his diaper and tried to feed him, to no avail. He screamed and cried, and no amount of consoling, burping, or anything else seemed to help. I started to cry, too.

A minute later, a woman came around the corner. She stood in front of the low-lit mirror fixing her hair and started a conversation with me through her reflection.

"I'm sorry, but I couldn't help overhearing your conversation," she said kindly. My mother and I had been discussing the checklist of interventions I tried.

"Oh, gosh, I'm so sorry . . ." I replied, immediately embarrassed and apologetic. She stopped me halfway through my sentence.

"No, no, don't apologize! That's not what I was going to say."

I relaxed and took a deep breath. It was hard enough to deal with an unhappy baby. I had nothing in me to deal with an unhappy stranger.

"Do you feed him formula by any chance?" she continued.

"I do sometimes, yes," I replied, interested, but fairly certain this would just be more guessing, or her telling me what a bad mom I was for doing that.

"Get him off the iron formula," she stated confidently. "My son had the exact same problem at that age. It took us weeks to figure it out. Formula is fortified with iron, but there's very little in breast milk. It can be extremely constipating for some babies, and it stopped the colic in its tracks when we removed it."

That afternoon my mom stayed with my son so I could go to the store to get some formula with low iron. When I returned, he had calmed down. He was lying on the floor on his play mat, and she was lying next to him rubbing his tummy.

"Julie, he has thrush," she said confidently. These women were so sure of themselves. I had no idea what that was.

"It's a yeast infection. Come here and look. I'll show you." I walked over, alarmed.

"See," she pointed inside his cheek. "That's thrush. Your brother had it."

She described my brother's case, which frightened me even more. My older brother had numerous health problems throughout his infancy: reflux, projectile vomiting, ear infections, bronchitis, pneumonia, and other problems. I panicked we were heading down the same path.

"The good news is it's very treatable," she said calmly. "Go call your doctor and get in there today. They can write you a script for an antifungal, and he'll be fine in a few days."

Within a few weeks of changing his formula and treating his thrush, and also after the nastiest, fluffiest, yellow poop I had ever seen, my son was back to normal. Sleep and healthy poop returned, and my baby was happy. It was true, I discovered. Breast milk contains very little iron.

The Homeland Security Act

It was never lost on me that my son's health returned at the hands of other moms. That episode was burned into my memory as the first time I realized other women could be more helpful than my doctors. I didn't articulate it in any way, but a sense of membership into some secret club, an underground railroad of mothers, washed over me. Moms knew, I learned that day. *Moms knew.*

I thought about that often as I read the message boards of the groups I joined to try to help Emma. Moms from all over the world were sharing their stories and theories of what troubled their children and what they were doing about it to help.

They talked about therapies and therapists, supplements and special diets, and environmental toxins. They discussed their favorite brands of fish oil, the best ways they found to document interventions, and so much more. They spoke a language I hadn't known existed and was intimidated yet anxious to learn. They really seemed to be helping their children.

But some of their theories, especially the vaccination one, still irritated me. I had completely forgotten about the correlation I made between Emma's illnesses and her developmental delays getting worse with each series of shots she received.

It had been years since she had any vaccines, and that no one ever mentioned them as a factor, especially her doctors, made me feel safe in my decision to give them to her. Honestly, I found myself with very little patience for those members of the group who kept bringing it up.

Delete. Delete. Delete.

That's the way I would deal with them. In my mind, it was irresponsible to suggest vaccines as a cause of developmental delay, not only for the guilt that could cause a parent, but also for the damage it could cause if everyone stopped vaccinating out of fear. Plus, didn't they know? The IOM proved it didn't happen.

And yet, a little voice about the wisdom of mothers, a subtle burning in my belly about what they knew and how, gave me pause. It was a mom who knew how to help my son. It was a mom in the office of the ear, nose, and throat specialist who told me about Early Intervention Services. It was my mom who recognized the thrush, and it was she, along with my mother-in-law, godmother, and grandmother, who insisted something was wrong with Emma.

It was always moms pointing me in the right direction. So why would they keep bringing it up? Why were so many of them convinced vaccines were an issue? What did they know that I didn't?

Truth be told, I never researched a vaccine in my life. I never even thought to. Vaccines to my generation were not just important, they were miraculous, arguably the greatest invention of mankind, responsible for saving the lives of countless millions.

For the first time ever, we were taught, man had outsmarted Mother Nature without meaningful consequence. Questioning vaccines was equivalent to questioning God, maybe worse. Lots of people my age questioned the existence of God. I didn't know a single person who questioned vaccines.

And then one day I saw it, a message about the Homeland Security Act. It drew me in if only for the fact that political posts were rare on the message boards I frequented. I read it just to see if it was a mistake. For a while I thought it was. The (paraphrased) post went something like this:

> At the eleventh hour, a rider nicknamed the "Lilly Rider" was inserted anonymously into the Homeland Security Act. This rider provided liability protection to pharmaceutical giant Eli Lilly for all potential lawsuits regarding their vaccine preservative Thimerosal. The rider was included in the passage of the act, however, at the outcry of parents, and in the absence of an author, was promptly removed thereafter.

I read the message several times. I had no idea what Thimerosal was or how it was remotely relevant to me, but this was weird. An anonymous legislator inserted a rider into the Homeland Security Act to grant federal protection from lawsuits to a pharmaceutical company for a vaccine ingredient? And then refused to come forward to defend it? Why?

Medicinal mercury

From then on, I scoured the Internet for information about Thimerosal. I learned it was an ethyl mercury–based preservative that was grandfathered into use prior to the existence of the FDA, and that Eli Lilly, in 1929 Indianapolis, conducted the only safety test on it before it was commercialized. They gave twenty-two adult patients with meningitis a 1 percent solution. All of them died. That was the safety study.

But before I learned any of the history of the product, I spent weeks trying to learn about mercury. I needed to know if it was possibly relevant to what was wrong with Emma. What did mercury do? What did mercury poisoning look like? How could you be exposed to it? What amount qualified as an overdose? Most important, how did you treat it?

At first I thought the answers would be very easy to find. That no one really knew that much about mercury, at least not compared to how much we were always warned and educated about lead, originally reassured me that it must be much safer. Going back to my baby bibles, I was reminded that the word *mercury* was nowhere to be found. This time I realized the word *autism* wasn't either.

Now, three years later, the absence of the words *mercury* and *autism* frightened me. The possibility I was stumbling upon an unexplored theory of causation was terrifying. If it was true, if this vaccine preservative was involved in making children sick, the consequences would be unfathomable.

I focused on learning about mercury. I reached out to friends and relatives in medical school or with chemistry majors who did their best to teach me. I even walked down to the chemistry teacher's classroom in the school where I taught and asked him for any texts, studies, or assistance he could offer.

Within a month, I had a library of information sprawled out on my dining room table. I learned exposure could be passed to the womb, and that according to the CDC, one in six women of child-bearing age was already considered mercury toxic enough to cause developmental harm to her child. I learned it was in our air, our soil, our oceans, our bodies, and our medicines.

I even learned from a student in a graduate class I taught that Thimerosal was controversial in animal vaccines. Way back in 1935, shortly after it had been patented, Pittman and Moore, an animal vaccine maker, determined it was too toxic for dogs. According to a letter written by the Director of Biological Services, "We have obtained marked local reaction in about 50% of the dogs injected with serum containing dilutions of Merthiolate (Thimerosal). Merthiolate is unsatisfactory as a preservative for serum intended for use on dogs."

Even so, it was used in contact lens solution and other ophthalmological products. And I also learned that it was in the silver fillings in my mouth. I remembered needing an emergency root canal on one when I was five months pregnant with Emma. I had completely forgotten about that.

My teeth. My womb. My air. My food. My contacts. My medicine. My milk. This poison, this horrific, deadly, awful toxin that could cause a loss of the ability to speak, tremors, memory loss, hallucinations, sleep disturbances, muscle cramps, constipation, rashes, tooth loss, and so much more . . . this horrific, deadly, awful toxin that I had known nothing about less than two months before . . . surrounded me.

It was everywhere, and yet we lived and acted as if it were nowhere and did nothing. That plume of smoke 5.2 miles from my house to the west, the same plume I saw rising in the sky since moving there in 1979, that plume was mercury. Poison floating over my house.

Those ugly silver fillings, the thirteen of them I had, were made up in part of the same poison. The contacts my mother and brother had worn their entire lives, and that I started wearing right around 1992, were soaked in poison, too.

The red dye in Mike's tattoo also contained mercury. And there were countless other products my parents and loved ones had been exposed to that contained it, including a very old tube of mercurochrome my dad kept in his bathroom drawer to put on his cuts for as long as I could remember.

From the second floor of our home, particularly from the window of the nursery, I could see the coal-burning plant off in the distance. The familiar symbol of my hometown had suddenly morphed from a landmark to a weapon against mankind. It wasn't bad enough that I had a sick child, I would think as I stared at it in horror. We have a sick planet, and the mercury pollution spewed over us, a by-product of burning coal, is a big reason why.

Every day, I anguished, I was breathing in mercury, running in it, swimming in it, existing in it. It was one of many ways I was no longer able to look at the world around me the way I once had. Nothing, and I mean nothing, would ever be the same.

Sinister synergy

While I researched, I was completely unaware of the controversy surrounding Thimerosal that had gone on for years. Because we didn't have a diagnosis when I first heard of it, and because I spent the majority of my time in speech-delay chat rooms, I came to it with the perspective of a skeptical outsider. It forced me to learn everything about mercury on my own, draw my own conclusions, and research independently of other parents. I am forever grateful for that, as no one influenced me.

By the spring of 2005, it was official; my daughter had autism. We finally had a diagnosis. But besides behavioral therapy, it seemed there wasn't much you could do. Mainstream medicine had little to offer us in terms of treatment or guidance, either. One of my friends was actually told to just take her son fishing.

And yet, many people, including a United States senator, believed mainstream medicine was wrong, and more important, potentially responsible for causing autism in the first place. It sounded crazy, but as I investigated, I could see why he believed it. Every single thing that was wrong with Emma could be explained at least in part by mercury poisoning, from the repeated illnesses, to the loss of skills, to the staring spells, to the head shaking—everything.

I also knew that she had been exposed to mercury in her vaccines. In 1997, following an act by the Food and Drug Administration (FDA) to tally up the amount of mercury still used in medicinal products, the Centers for Disease Control (CDC) discovered they had not calculated the total amount of mercury children could be exposed to in their vaccines when they added two new vaccines to the recommended schedule in the early 1990s that contained it.

By adding these vaccines to the recommended schedule, the amount of mercury exposure a baby could have not only almost tripled in amount, but also moved up to the day of birth. If it turned out to be problematic, it would arguably be one of the most catastrophic oversight errors ever.

All of the involved regulatory agencies were panicked at the prospect they had done something horrible, and by 1999, when neither the FDA nor the CDC had made a public statement about it, the American Academy of Pediatrics acted on its own to do just that.

In the summer of 1999, on a Friday afternoon when almost no one was paying attention, they called for an end to mercury's use in vaccines, even though they did not request a recall. It was a confusing and contradictory position at best. On the one hand, they were admitting it could be a serious problem, but on the other, they were not immediately taking it all off the shelves.

Regardless of the statement, the FDA never issued a ban, and much of the product remained on the shelves for years until it ran out. It was entirely plausible that Emma received whatever was still around in early 2001. And in 2004, inexplicably, they added annual flu shots to the recommended vaccine schedule for pregnant women and babies six months of age and older, many of which contained the same full dose of mercury simultaneously being phased out in other vaccines. Contrary to the common belief that mercury was eliminated from use in vaccines, it was far from gone.

I grabbed her vaccine records and compared the lot numbers and manufacturers to the information I found on a CDC website. Indeed, more than two years after the American Academy of Pediatrics had worried enough to call a press conference for mercury's discontinued use, Emma had been exposed to a small dose of it in some of her vaccines. I ran to the bathroom and almost became sick to my stomach.

I wanted to cry, but I couldn't, and I wanted to scream, but I couldn't do that, either. My whole body felt frozen, thoughts swirling in my mind of my root canal and holding Emma down to be injected with this toxin after being given not only antibiotics and aluminum-containing vaccines, but also acetaminophen. Acetaminophen, most commonly known as Tylenol, is now widely accepted as being dangerous to a baby, partly because it impairs the body's ability to excrete toxins. Giving it to Emma before and after her vaccines that contained mercury and aluminum was a terrible mistake.

One of the researchers whose work I had been reading while I investigated mercury made it clear what had likely happened to Emma. Dr. Boyd Haley, Chemistry Professor Emeritus and Department Chair of the University of Kentucky, who specializes in mercury toxicity, described what could have happened based on an experiment he did.

According to Dr. Haley, if you expose brain tissue to the same amount and type of aluminum that is found in vaccines (aluminum is used to provoke an immune response), the aluminum had almost no toxic effect on the neurons; however, Thimerosal caused the neurons to start dying.

But more alarmingly, he also found that when you combined the aluminum and Thimerosal, it was six to ten times more toxic. Aluminum and mercury had a synergistic effect. It confirmed the precaution listed on the Material Safety Data Sheet for Thimerosal, which clearly states Thimerosal should never be combined with aluminum for this very reason.

Likewise, he discovered, there were other confounding factors. For example, it has been known for decades that antibiotics also enhance the toxicity of Thimerosal. As far back as the early 1970s, women who wore contact lenses and used a solution that contained Thimerosal were not allowed to wear them when being treated for a urinary tract infection because the antibiotic tetracycline dramatically enhanced the toxicity of Thimerosal.

Sure enough, when he did the same experiment with antibiotics, the same thing happened. When he exposed the neurons from the brain tissue in culture to antibiotics, there was little effect. Once again, however, and as expected, when the antibiotics were combined with Thimerosal, the toxicity was dramatically enhanced. He often reiterated his serious concerns while speaking on the matter:

> Many times, when I've been talking to parents who have two or three children, and even identical twins or twins, one of

> them autistic and one of them not . . . the one that was autistic was also the one who had ear infections and was given antibiotics, as well as the vaccines, during the well-baby visits.
>
> So I think it's something that really needs to be studied. I think there is absolutely no doubt, from animal studies, that antibiotics dramatically enhance the retention and uptake of mercury into the body and enhance the toxicity of mercury exposure, Thimerosal as well.

The hypothesis made perfect sense. Emma had been exposed to mercury as a baby in my womb from my root canal and air pollution, and she was on antibiotics from the moment she was born, over ten rounds of them in the first two years of her life. She was also very likely sensitive to aluminum like her father and grandfather, both of whom have significant reactions to anything with aluminum. (Neither her father nor grandfather can wear aluminum-containing antiperspirants without breaking out into a horrific rash.)

She was then repeatedly injected with aluminum- and mercury-containing vaccines *while on antibiotics and Tylenol*, the combination and amount of which had finally manifested as brain damage.

She presented with the symptoms of mercury poisoning, so perhaps she actually had mercury poisoning. It had to be that—or I was disappointed in her, or she had some rare genetic condition not found on either side of our family that had yet to be identified that manifested exactly the same way.

That I had possibly done this to her . . . that I was responsible . . . that I had failed to protect her . . . and that those I depended on had failed to protect us both . . . it was too much to take.

I slumped against the wall in disbelief. I had not yet remembered that I also occasionally breastfed her while eating canned tuna once or twice a week for a few weeks, and I wouldn't remember for five more years.

Autism begins to speak

Later that month, NBC launched a weeklong program dedicated to autism. Bob Wright, the president of NBC, had a grandchild with autism, and he wanted to bring awareness to the burgeoning epidemic. The numbers were staggering. Estimates were that 1 in 68 families had a child diagnosed with autism. Something had to be done.

As happy as everyone online was to see the issue getting attention, the majority of the chatroom messages were angry for two main reasons. One, NBC kept calling autism a purely genetic disorder. And two, nothing about Thimerosal or mercury was mentioned. One night on the *Nightly News* with Brian Williams, as he tried to address the angry emails he had been flooded with, a doctor dismissed their concerns that autism was a man-made disorder caused by vaccination as "an old wives' tale" that hadn't been proven.

It was true that it hadn't been "proven" by the handful of population studies recently published by the CDC and reviewed by the IOM. But those studies were fraught with flaws.

For example, they had compared the rates of autism among children exposed to small amounts of vaccine mercury with those who had been exposed to more and reported they couldn't determine if there was a problem. Nonetheless, it was included as part of the evidence to dismiss the hypothesis of a potential link.

More importantly, the studies weren't biologically based. There were many things that could prove a link biologically, such as chelating. Chelating is the standard medical procedure for removing heavy metals from the body. By using a substance called a "chelator" that is able to grab the metal and carry it out of the body, mercury can be expelled from a person. Depending on the source of exposure, coupled with whether or not there is chronic or acute poisoning, chelators may be given intravenously, transdermally, or orally.

Regardless of protocol, and although some chelators are available over the counter, chelation should be practiced under the guidance of a physician. It can be dangerous, and in a tragic event that gave the practice a bad name for years to come, the wrong chelator was once given to a child by his physician that caused his death.

Even so, in early 2005, some parents were reporting that their children going through chelation were losing their autism diagnosis as the mercury came out. According to them, their children were recovering. Didn't that prove a link?

The media presented a story about chelation, calling it a risky procedure being used by desperate parents. It focused on a boy who was chelated at age two and had legitimately recovered. The same regional center that had diagnosed him with autism was the same regional center that determined he no longer had autism. The parents needed no convincing of what happened. Mercury went in, boy got sick. Mercury came out, boy got better. Where was the controversy?

The expert asked to comment had a simple explanation. According to her, the boy never had autism to begin with. Apparently his parents and doctors had been mistaken. It sounded stupid, but it was an important comment, I felt. Mercury poisoning could be mistaken for autism. She just said so.

Newsweek also did a story on autism. Suddenly, this condition that was never mentioned anywhere in the 600 pages of my 1994 edition of *Caring for Your Baby and Child: Birth to Age Five* was everywhere. Mercury, however, was not.

There was no mention that autism had not been discovered until the late 1930s, approximately seven years after Thimerosal was commercialized. There was no mention that Thimerosal had nearly tripled in exposure at the beginning of the early 1990s with the addition of two new vaccines to the childhood recommended vaccine schedule.

No mention was included that no one had ever added up the cumulative amount of mercury being injected as shots, or that a memo leaked to the *Los Angeles Times* confirmed that Merck knew in 1991 that kids could be getting up to eighty-seven times the amount of mercury exposure based on what was safe for an adult but did nothing.

No mention that Thimerosal can separate and sink to the bottom of a vaccine vial if not shaken vigorously as directions indicate, which could lead to a larger dose than what was expected. (This meant that the epidemiological studies on its safety were using theoretical exposure rates only. Even today, we do not know the exact amount individuals have been exposed to.)

No mention that mercury and testosterone are synergistic, which makes the vaccines much more dangerous for boys, or that autism affects four times as many boys than girls. No mention that it is synergistic with aluminum, either, or that it is often administered with aluminum-containing vaccines, even though it clearly states on the material safety data sheet that the two should never be combined.

The list went on. What the media and medicine were telling us was that Thimerosal, made up of almost 50 percent ethyl mercury, could not and did not cause the symptoms of autism, virtually identical to the symptoms of mercury poisoning—so close, in fact, that a boy had been misdiagnosed.

Mercury cannot cause mercury poisoning, they claimed; attempting to prove it by removing mercury from a body was dangerous; and if it worked, it was only a coincidence.

Emails urging everyone to share his or her story with Representative Dan Burton, a Republican from Indiana, kept coming. He wanted to collect piles of stories from parents across the country to make a point to the federal government. He was a champion of the cause, along with Congressman Dave Weldon of Florida, a medical doctor. Burton had an autistic grandchild. He was convinced mercury was responsible.

There was also a father featured on an MSNBC program that month named J. B. Handley who was speaking out. In a calm, matter-of-fact manner, he identified mercury as the culprit behind his son's regression into autism. He also mentioned that he and his wife were about to launch a new organization to help parents and their affected kids. It was called Generation Rescue and would be up the first week of March.

And there was something else according to one of the messages on the boards. There was a book coming out April 1. It was called *Evidence of Harm: Mercury in Vaccines and the Autism Epidemic: A Medical Controversy*, written by a journalist named David Kirby.

A book? I thought, flabbergasted, when I learned about it. I had been investigating autism for some time and never heard a word. *How long had everyone known about this?* I wondered.

The answer was eight years. In November 1997, following the call of the Food and Drug Administration Modernization Act, the government began to do the math. And what they calculated wasn't good. They could appear to have been "asleep at the switch" when allowing two new Thimerosal vaccines to be added to the childhood vaccination schedule in the early 1990s.

It was the very reason the American Academy of Pediatrics had held a press conference to call for its removal. Contrary to what frequently gets reported, it was the government, not parents, that first discovered what they had done.

April, the Amish, and some monkeys

In addition to David Kirby's book, April 2005 presented itself as the month lines would be drawn in the sand: "Parents versus Research," the *New York Times* would later call it. Although the controversy had raged quietly behind the scenes for several years, it was now getting national and mainstream attention.

The month of media coverage in February, the launch of autism advocacy organizations Autism Speaks and Generation Rescue shortly thereafter, and now the release of a study on the toxicity of ethyl mercury were charging full speed ahead.

A scientist named Thomas Burbacher had produced an important study on Thimerosal. Thimerosal is ethyl mercury, a form of the toxin created by the scientist Morris Kharasch, a Ukrainian immigrant and chemical engineer. He had been recruited by the US government to help create chemical weapons in response to Germany's use of them in World War I.

He synthesized a new form of mercury, one that was designed to be a "targeted toxin." Although mercury was accepted as highly toxic, the prevailing thought was that the right use of it in the right form administered the right way would allow man to harness its toxicity to destroy the bad while not hurting the good. We still believe this is possible, and it's the justification for its use in vaccines to this day.

He took his new mercury with him to the University of Chicago after the war was over. There, he sold the patent to commercialize it into three products: a biological preservative, a lumber preservative, and a seed preservative. The seed and lumber preservatives were eventually banned for being too toxic. However, the biological preservative, Thimerosal, is still used in vaccines and other products today.

Burbacher was studying the differences between Kharasch's "targeted toxin" and the more commonly known methyl mercury. Methyl mercury is the form found in fish, and it is the form on which all of our current exposure guidelines are based. This study set out to see if that had been a responsible thing to do. If Thimerosal was more toxic and also being injected, rather than ingested, we did not have accurate safety guidelines.

Burbacher injected monkeys with both kinds of organic mercury. Upon analysis, he discovered ethyl mercury behaved differently than methyl mercury in a body. It left the blood faster than methyl mercury, which initially seemed to imply it would be safer, but it was not. Ethyl mercury, it turned out, went to the brain faster than methyl mercury. There, it got trapped in larger amounts as inorganic mercury. Any inorganic mercury in a brain is extremely dangerous and toxic. That ethyl mercury accelerated and intensified that possibility was extraordinary. These findings were significant.

The message boards were buzzing. The CDC's studies to exonerate Thimerosal thus far had been population based, and they had been using theoretical exposure rates. And the IOM didn't rely exclusively on biological studies to exonerate it either, even though in 2001 they claimed the theory was biologically plausible. Oddly, they were dismissing a biologically plausible theory without relying on biology.

Not only that, looking at their population studies carefully exposed questionable study practices, highly stratified data, and conclusions that indicated that high levels of exposure to this neurotoxin had a *protective* effect. In other words, their science was suggesting Thimerosal could prevent autism. Their illogical scientific conclusions and suspicious behavior were the central concern of David Kirby's book.

Now there was an animal study that showed Thimerosal was dangerous to a brain. It didn't prove Thimerosal caused autism, but it proved there was a problem, and it proved that using methyl mercury guidelines to determine its danger was wrong.

We waited for the news reports to confirm our concerns. Before any appeared, Representative Dave Weldon, the doctor from Florida, fired off a letter to the National Institutes of Health demanding answers. He even issued a press release. There had always been a lot of smoke surrounding this issue. Now there was fire.

I remember sitting in my office chair turned toward the television behind me as an anchor came on to tell us the news. Anxious to hear the report, I hung on her every word. Unfortunately, it was not what I had hoped for.

"A new study has confirmed that ethyl mercury remains in the blood for less time than methyl mercury," she reported seriously. "It turns out, it's actually less dangerous than we thought."

My mouth dropped at the manipulative statement. It was true that it left the blood earlier, yes, but that was because it went to the brain and stayed there! Either she hadn't understood the study or she was purposefully misreporting the study. I couldn't figure out which was worse.

The information about ethyl mercury's history, the story of Morris Kharasch and Thimerosal's sister products, remained unknown to most of us for several years. It was then that journalist Dan Olmsted and a colleague of his, Mark Blaxill, the father of an affected child, presented this evidence in their groundbreaking book, *The Age of Autism: Mercury, Medicine, and a Man-Made Epidemic*.

But in April 2005, none of us parents had ever heard of Dan. We didn't know that he was responsible for reporting on the dangers of an anti-malaria medication given to soldiers that was causing psychological problems, or that because of his reporting it would be labeled as being potentially dangerous. We didn't know he went to Yale, or that he was one of the original staff members of *USA Today*. We would come to learn all of this later.

All we knew was that seemingly out of the blue, he started writing a series of articles for United Press International about autism. And Dan had a question.

He wanted to know if the Amish, who are known not to vaccinate, had autism. If they didn't experience autism at the same rate as the vaccinating population, it could be an important clue.

He was determined to investigate and wrote an article that would change his life forever. The answer was no. The Amish did not have autism in their unvaccinated children as far as he could find.

Chapter 7

Treatment—Blood on My Hands

About a month after the appointment with the neurologist who suggested we see a family therapist to overcome our disappointment in Emma, we had our first appointment with a medical doctor who specialized in autism spectrum disorders. He was our second choice; the one we had hoped to see had an eight-month waiting list.

Upon being told that her problems were likely the result of my husband and me being disappointed in her, or that we were somehow making them worse by being mad at her, I was done messing around. I decided to go straight to the leading autism expert in the country, Dr. Bernard Rimland.

Dr. Rimland was the father of an affected child, and more importantly, he was the man who challenged and changed the paradigm that "disappointed" mothers had anything to do with causing autism. I already loved him for that.

Since the early 1940s when autism was first discovered, mothers had been blamed for causing it, which I hadn't known. Psychiatry at that time was still heavily influenced by the ideas of Sigmund Freud that had to do with the power of a parent to cause a mental disorder in his or her child. As evidence, the doctor to eventually give autism a name, Dr. Leo Kanner, hypothesized that cold, uncaring mothers caused their children to turn inward for the love they didn't receive. Unbeknownst to me, that had remained the prevailing theory for almost fifty years.

At the time, however, he was on the other side of the country. Although I was happy to get on a plane the next day if necessary, I was informed there were other specialists in the country besides him who could help. I was given a few recommendations and decided to see the first available.

My godmother went with me as she promised she would do at Thanksgiving. It was nice to have the company, but it was more important to have the extra ears and instinct. My mind was flooded with questions, chemistry, and anxiety. Although I brought a notebook to take notes, I was grateful for another person to hear what the doctor would say.

It was somewhat disappointing. I wanted to get started helping her on the spot, but that would not be the case. We had testing to do first, he insisted, and lots of it. It would take several weeks to get the results, and it wouldn't be until afterward that he would give me any specific guidance on how to move forward.

I was crushed. My patience was wearing thin, but all was not lost. This doctor had a lot to offer. Unlike the neurologist, he went over her medical history in detail. He was also the father of a child on the spectrum. He spent over an hour with us, conducting tests and asking questions, and seemed genuinely interested in Emma's well-being and in helping her feel better. Most importantly, he didn't seem the least bit inclined to blame me.

"She's on the spectrum for sure," he confirmed at the end, going into more detail on the severity and the type he believed it was. Although I was happy to finally have the diagnosis, and would have it confirmed elsewhere shortly thereafter by a second specialist we had also been waiting to see, I was uncomfortable with it.

She was clearly a sick little girl who needed medical treatment. Saying otherwise was a lie, and I was not about to dishonor her truth. How in the world autism could be considered a *mental* disorder was beyond me. Eczema? Repeated illnesses? Low muscle tone? Drooling? The loss of the ability to speak? Sleeping problems? Constipation? Did they think she was making herself sick? We weren't imagining any of this!

We left with a prescription for blood work, a few test kits to check other metabolic issues and co-morbid conditions, and some suggested dietary restrictions. My aunt, who had a background in psychology, agreed with his assessment but didn't offer much else. Her confidence reassured me we were on the right path but also concerned me. It was the absence of dissenting opinion and information that had led me here to begin with.

At home, I placed the kits on the counter in the order I needed to complete them and began reading through the packet of dietary information he provided. As hard as I tried not to, I felt overwhelmed. There was so much to do and learn. Every time I thought we took one step forward, I felt pushed three or four steps back. Every time I thought I had a grasp on what to do and why, I became more confused.

To stay focused, in the dining room–turned–library, I created a new journal. Instead of documenting her illnesses and developmental delays as I had been, I needed to start documenting test results and interventions.

I created a form to keep track of what she could eat; how and when she pooped; her overall health; what interventions we used that day; and any behavior, speech, or progress of note. From that day forward for the next several years, I filled it out religiously. It provided me with tremendous evidence of improvement down the road.

Gluten-free, casein-free

From what I remember, the theory went like this: a gut that was inflamed or damaged, perhaps by the overgrowth of yeast and bad bacteria, could become permeable and allow undigested food to seep into the bloodstream. Two of those undigested proteins found most commonly in wheat and dairy products, gluten and casein, happened to mimic opioids.

Hypothetically, they could fill opioid receptors, thereby leading a child to look like he or she was high. It could potentially explain the dazed-out, strung-out, absent look in the eyes of many affected children.

By 2005, many parents were testing this theory on their own. Of the maybe four books on autism I could find anywhere that year, two dealt with treating it through diet and digestive enzymes. One mom went so far as to consider her child recovered by the diet. It was certainly worth a try.

But "try" turned out to be the operative word. In early 2005, trying to find gluten-free foods was difficult at best. Finding gluten- and casein-free foods was nearly impossible.

In the grocery store, I walked the aisles in a daze. This familiar place I had shopped since I was a teenager felt foreign. Another part of my once-comfortable life had become a stressor. Gone were the days of running into the store to grab some milk, bread, and dinner for the evening. It took forever to read all of the boxes.

Now everything had to be investigated, researched, checked, and double-checked for safe ingredients. According to the moms on the message boards, if you didn't commit to the diet 100 percent, you were wasting your time and money. Even one small bite of a cracker was enough to ruin everything for days, they claimed.

So I searched and searched for safe foods. Our choices were limited to fresh fruits and vegetables, chicken breast, beef, potatoes, eggs, rice milk, and a handful of existing gluten-free snacks that were placed on a small shelf at the back of the store. Most of them tasted disgusting.

It quickly became clear that I was going to have to do most of the food preparation and cooking myself in order to accommodate

Emma's needs. There were some flours I could buy if I wanted to make my own bread, something I needed to do after tasting the only one on the market. Now I was not only in charge of figuring out what had happened to my daughter and learning how to treat it, I also had to become a baker and a chef.

I stared at the few products on the gluten-free shelf in grief and fear. I grabbed the little bag of gluten-free flour, turned it over to check for casein, and surrendered to the tremendous need I had to sit down. In complete defeat, in the middle of the aisle, I did just that.

Blood on my hands

Within two months of our diagnosis, we had spent several thousand dollars out of pocket on medical testing and treatment, private therapy, organic food, supplements, and more. Autism was and still is considered a psychiatric condition. Insurance plans would not cover much beyond psychiatric medication. Everything was out of pocket.

Instead, parents seeking medical treatment for their affected children, who were trying to eliminate the underlying co-morbid conditions autism presented to see if it would help, were left to fill out the insurance paperwork and hope. For example, if we wanted to try a specific medical treatment that wasn't necessarily covered under an autism diagnosis, we had no choice but to submit the claim for insurance afterward and see if we qualified for reimbursement. It was yet another thing to deal with, and it usually didn't help anyway. Almost nothing we submitted to our insurance plan was reimbursed.

Such was the case with the blood panel that was ordered after the initial test results came back, something that would cost even more money. We still had to complete the blood work from the kits that had come home with us, and now we needed to do more.

To get it all done at once, I chose a day that I could get home from school earlier than usual. Emma had to fast until the blood draw, and I didn't want to keep her waiting any longer than was necessary. We arrived at the suggested lab, I feeling anxious, she feeling hungry. I was not looking forward to holding her down again.

At the lab, I was told they would not be able to do the blood work for the kits. In spite of what our doctor told us, I would have to get that blood drawn at a hospital, and most likely by appointment. I agreed to let them draw the blood for the panel anyway and had no choice but to do the kits another time. We went home and finally got Emma something to eat.

My frustration and disappointment by then were palpable, the amount of hoops I had to jump through for so long constantly tripping me up. Without realizing it yet, I was at my boiling point.

Although it had technically only been a few weeks since the diagnosis, it had been years of being dismissed by doctors, watching my daughter disappear before my eyes, being accused of not paying attention to her or being disappointed in her, researching what could be wrong, being put on waiting lists, and so much more that brought me to the brink.

Now that we finally had an answer and a direction, my patience for any more setbacks or roadblocks was gone. Anyone or anything in my way needed to watch out. I wanted to fix autism, fix it now, and be done with it. I had nothing left in me to accommodate incompetence. Incompetence had cost my daughter enough already.

At the hospital a few days later, a new phlebotomist worked a miracle. Having her blood drawn was still fresh in her mind, and Emma's cooperation was initially poor. This young woman did an amazing job of helping her relax, getting her to laugh, and getting the blood she needed. I was relieved to finally be able to put this behind us.

As we were leaving, she asked if we needed to spin the blood. I had no idea, and did not know why that would be necessary. I hadn't read her instructions, only mine, so I asked her to check. A few seconds later, as if realizing she had asked something foolish, she exhaled relieved, and packed up the box without spinning anything. She handed me the kit with a smile, tussled Emma's hair while complimenting her for being such a good girl, and reminded me that the sample had to be kept cold.

At home I called FedEx for a pickup, but while placing the items into the envelope provided, realized something was wrong. Several tubes included in the kit had not been used. I had done enough kits by then to know that wasn't right. They didn't come with extras.

Panicking, I pulled out the contents to double-check everything. I finally read the technician's instructions, something I hadn't considered prior. I had to be a phlebotomist now, too?

Sure enough, according to the directions, she was supposed to spin the blood. Not only that, she was supposed to mix it with whatever was in the other tubes. Worse, it had to be done within fifteen minutes to be of any use.

It was for nothing. All of it had been for nothing. The babysitter I paid for two days in one week. The time off of work. The stress. The tears. The hunger. The cost. For nothing. I lost it.

"Goddamn it!" I shouted, even though all of my children were in the kitchen with me. "Damn them! Damn them! Damn them! Damn them!"

One of the children, startled by my crazed reaction, asked what was wrong.

"They messed it up! Those stupid fuckers messed it up!"

"Julie!" Mike scolded me furiously. "Enough! Relax!"

"Oh, shut up, Mike! Just shut up!" I shouted back. I was not about to let him, or anyone, tell me how to feel or react. He had no idea what this had been like, in my mind.

Desperate and angry, I attempted to spin the blood and mix the tubes myself. I knew it was insane to try, but in my panic and rage, I couldn't let this all go to waste. Maybe, just maybe, I could make it right.

I frantically rolled the tube of blood between my hands like two sticks being used to start a fire, as if that could even come close to the actual spinning that takes place in the centrifuge, and opened the cap with a pop. Her blood popped out all over with it.

On the envelope, on the kit, on the table, on my shirt, on my face, and all over my hands was Emma's splattered blood. I stood in despair and disbelief; the horror of how I felt on the inside now manifested in the world around me on the outside. Emma's blood was literally on my hands, and I had terrorized my family in the process.

Pretty accurate, I would think.

Disney 2.0

It was supposed to be the happiest place on earth. Three years prior when we took our son for the first time, it still was. Although we left Emma behind that year due to her age and repeated illness, Disney World still felt magical then. I always loved Disney and couldn't wait to share that experience with all of my children.

And so in the summer of 2005, we decided to treat the family as we had planned, this time with Emma. She may not remember this trip, I realized, but I would. The thought of getting her a little princess dress, taking pictures with the characters, and visiting Cinderella's castle had once made my heart soar. I envisioned our time there together since she was born. Capturing those images and memories was on my parent bucket list.

But as the trip approached, anxiety clutched my chest. Autism was stealing everything from me by the day. In addition to taking my daughter, it was taking my reality, my time, my money, my profession, my trust, my sleep, my confidence, my dreams, and even, I worried, my marriage.

In only the few short months that we had been diagnosed, everything about our life had changed—where we could eat, what we could eat, where we could go, when we could go, and how we could spend our time.

My time was almost entirely dedicated to autism. It was all I could think about, all I could concentrate on. Honestly, it was all I wanted to think about. The world inside my computer, where like-minded parents, physicians, journalists, activists, and politicians spent their time and energy on email threads and chat groups, was the only world where I wanted to be. In there, I was safe. I was invigorated. I was learning. I could *do* something. *I had to do something.*

The kids, our home, my career, and my husband came second, third, fourth, and fifth in that order. Nothing mattered as much as learning everything I could to help my little girl, making the connections with the people that could also help, and stopping this from happening to anyone else.

There was a rally about mercury and autism taking place in Washington, DC, the week we were in Orlando. I was truly torn about where I should be and even considered leaving Mike and the kids in Disney to attend it. I didn't.

But in Disney World, the magic had escaped. Where I once felt inspired and childlike, I now felt cautious and out of place. Like the grocery store, like the water park, like the doctor's office, it morphed into a dangerous place.

Emma could get lost or hurt anywhere here. The lights and sights and sounds overwhelmed her. It took only one time on the It's a Small World ride to realize rides like that were a mistake. The loud repetitive song coupled with the weird moving figures in the dark frightened her deeply. She held her hands over her ears the whole time and mostly kept her eyes closed. Afterward, we carefully navigated our way through stores and eliminated rides that could cause her potential pain.

For me, however, it became impossible. Everywhere was pain. Healthy children surrounded me. Babbling toddlers and ice cream cones she couldn't have bombarded me visually. And without access to my computer, with no smartphones yet, I felt isolated from the only people who understood my heartbreak or me. Disney, I realized, was a disaster.

But it wasn't about me, I told myself daily. I would create these memories, damn it, no matter what it took. We bought that princess dress. We went to Cinderella's castle, and, disregarding the weeks we had spent dedicated to the diet, I bought her an ice cream cone from the iconic parlor on Main Street. We swam in the pool, watched the fireworks while I covered her ears, and went on all of the rides she could tolerate.

Except for the teacups. I would not go on them or anything that had to do with Alice in Wonderland. Mad Hatters, I learned, were called that because they had gone crazy from mercury poisoning. Felt hats used to be treated with mercury. I was not about to do anything with my daughter that hinted that mercury poisoning was fun or entertaining. For us, it was nothing short of a nightmare.

Orlando baked in the summer sun, and most days we set out early to explore the parks before we overheated. One morning while in the Magic Kingdom, Emma pointed to the Dumbo ride. It went around in circles, gently lifting up and down as it did. I contemplated whether it would be too much for her while she pulled me toward the line. Apparently she didn't think so.

Behind us a couple stood with their teenaged daughter. She made subtle unintelligible noises while looking closely at her fingers. She didn't say a word, nor did her parents, as we waited for over twenty minutes.

As much as I desperately wanted to start a conversation, I feared I would offend or hurt them by doing so. I knew I had tried to come to Disney World to escape talking about or thinking about autism. I imagined they did the same. I was still naïve and hopeful enough to believe that was possible.

In our elephant, Emma looked around with glee. I memorized her face as her blonde hair blew behind her, the castle, other rides, and some shops circling by. Even though I desperately tried not to, I couldn't help but think of the young girl behind us with her parents.

Was she enjoying the ride? I wondered. It was impossible to tell. *Was this Emma's fate?* I panicked. *Would they be us in ten years?*

We got off the ride, and I asked her if she had fun. Despite the few words she had, she could not fully express how she felt. From her happy expression and nodding yes to my question, I could tell that she had a great time, but my heart burned for her and the other girl that they could not tell us in their own words. I prayed that she would remember, and that even if she could never express herself completely, she could hold these memories dear.

I knelt down to hug her and noticed she was very warm. Emma's body didn't regulate temperature well, and even though it was still morning, she was sweating and flushed. I spotted the shops we circled past and headed in one to cool her off in the air conditioning.

In the candy store, I bought her a humungous lollipop. *To hell with the diet,* I argued internally. *We're on vacation. Treatment is, too.*

We have to move

My struggle to maintain a normal life had intensified by the end of summer. In my original life plan, we would build a dream house in our late thirties or early forties when I went back to work after staying home with the kids for many years. My future income would provide us with the ability to send them to college without debt, secure a nice pension, take vacations, and allow us to build our own home.

But just as Emma's health had presented a change in plans, as we decided it was best for me to continuing teaching to provide better insurance and pay for private therapy, so had the housing market.

Although we hadn't been thinking about moving, we now felt pressured to do so immediately. If we didn't move soon, we worried, we would never be able to. Not only had our house almost doubled in value since we had purchased it six years earlier, new construction was skyrocketing in cost. It felt like it was now or never.

More importantly, just steps away from our patio doors was an above-ground pool surrounded by a deck. It was one of the main features of the home that I loved when we purchased it. I had a pool growing up, and it held some of my fondest childhood memories. After Emma escaped from the hotel room, I started hating it.

At the top of the doors there were locks to make sure the kids could never get outside without our help, but I knew it would only take once for someone to leave the door unlocked accidentally for something awful to happen. Horror stories of children with autism eloping at night, wandering away from family parties, and even setting their homes on fire were now a part of the news cycle.

Two brothers with autism in a neighboring suburb had burned down their home. Several months earlier, another child had wandered off and froze to death. It was becoming widely known that children with autism who wandered were drawn to water. There was a death trap fifteen feet from our kitchen table.

Worse, we lived on a busy corner. One of the streets did not yet have a stop sign, and the other street, straight and wide, allowed cars to speed along at over forty miles per hour by the time they reached us.

In our backyard, our pool was a threat. In our front yard, our neighbors' cars were. Nowhere felt safe. We signed a contract with a local builder and moved six months later after living with my parents for a few months.

All of the distractions—my obsession with everything autism; building a new home; going back to work full time; treating Emma medically, behaviorally, and otherwise; trying to maintain some normalcy; trying to maintain our marriage—all of these things I was doing in an attempt to give myself the life I always wanted, and always wanted to provide for my family, distracted me from the significance of something else that was happening.

Treating Emma was working. By the time we moved in December, she no longer qualified for Early Intervention Services.

Chapter 8

Recovery—Why Do Elephants Eat Grass?

It was the same room as the year prior when we had been evaluated to see if she qualified for Early Intervention Services through the school district when she turned three years old. The same bench I had sat on praying she would have a friend and be like the other little girls marching in front of me was still in the same hallway.

The same posters decorated the same yellow cement block walls. The same rug for reading time with the same beanbag chairs and the same bookshelves remained in the back corner. And the same tables, one rectangular and one kidney-bean shaped, both low to the ground for children, stood near opposite walls.

Last time I had sat at the rectangular one. At it, I was told Emma was zoning out, in need of occupational and physical therapy, and significantly verbally and cognitively impaired. At that table, I first experienced what it felt like to have strangers rattle off skills that my child could not demonstrate, listing them respectfully but clinically with a smile, using careful language to make it sound like what she could do was positive even though the overall picture was not.

This would be what an Individualized Education Plan (IEP) would feel like, I learned that day. An emotional war zone where verbal daggers disguised as compliments and concern sank deep into your chest faster than you could process or realize.

You spent the whole time ducking and weaving, listening to the problems your child presented and the interventions the school was willing to implement, trying not to sink or explode with despair, trying to concentrate and document their words, and trying to figure out whether the school was genuinely crafting a plan of action for what was best or only for what they could afford. Lots of parents believed it was the latter. It is no coincidence there is always a box of tissues in the middle of the table.

Long before I had children, I had studied IEPs while preparing to be a teacher. By law, all schools must provide students with disabilities and special education needs with an opportunity to learn in the least restrictive environment.

Schools must also provide any therapies or interventions that students might need, such as speech and occupational therapy, psychological testing, or social work. Every year, parents, teachers, and therapists meet to go over the progress and plan of the year prior to determine how to move forward the next year. It is my absolute least favorite day of the year.

The year before, in the fall of 2004, at age three and a half, Emma had received a battery of tests to check her cognitive, social, and verbal abilities. In addition to the initial results from the transitional screening from the state's Early Intervention Services in the spring of that year, the school district's team of special education experts had determined Emma needed serious help.

By February 2005, she was placed in a special-needs preschool program. Since then, a little yellow bus had come to our house to pick her up to attend a half-day of school where she received all of the aforementioned therapies. She would then spend the afternoon in a regular preschool setting we paid for privately, followed by private therapy in our home.

The little bus frightened me not only for what it represented, but also for the fact my daughter was only three years old when she was on it alone with a stranger. It's hard enough to put a five-year-old on a bus full of neighborhood children when they head to kindergarten. Putting a three-year-old on it alone felt highly irresponsible, but with my work schedule, I had no choice.

To make matters worse, she also had to wear a complicated harness as a makeshift seat belt. With her limited verbal ability, I worried she wouldn't be able to tell the bus driver if anything went wrong or if she was uncomfortable. Buses could be very dangerous places because of that, I suspected. I hated that bus.

I sat stoic and straight-faced, taking deep breaths and going through my notes while waiting for the team of educators to join me. I flipped through the results of the year before to refresh my memory and began to wonder if she had met her goals for this year.

She must have, I believed. Emma had made incredible progress over the summer and early fall. I expected them to confirm my suspicions, create new goals, and be on my way. I did not expect what would actually happen.

The team finally came over to join me, all of us sitting in uncomfortable chairs that were too small for adults, forcing our knees up just a little too high and making us all look just a little ridiculous. Nonetheless, we continued as usual, the routine go-around of taking attendance, introducing new staff members, and exchanging pleasantries.

I took a deep breath, centered myself, and prepared for the emotional battle to come. It was good that I had. The director of services began with a shot out of a cannon.

"So, what have you been doing with Emma?" she asked curiously but not with a tone of wrongdoing. If anything, she was excited.

"I'm sorry?" I asked to buy some time. I was very cautious not to share anything about what we were doing outside the circle of people I trusted. Treating autism as a medical condition was considered radical at best, dangerous and irresponsible at worst. Even though I was working with two medical doctors and had a dossier of test results to confirm her medical issues, which were what I was actually treating, I was not about to tell the school district anything.

"You have to tell us what you've been doing," she continued looking around at the others nodding in agreement. "We've never seen anything like it."

I still had no idea what she was talking about. We were doing a lot of things besides medical interventions, from private preschool to private speech therapy, to physical therapy, to private tutoring, to play therapy, to reading programs. I assumed that must be what she meant.

"Mrs. Obradovic," she didn't let me respond. "These are Emma's test results from one year ago." She sprawled out the same papers as the ones I had in my possession.

"Here, she placed in the twentieth percentile," she pointed to one skill. "And here, she's in the tenth," she pointed to another. She reiterated all of Emma's social and verbal limitations from that time.

"And here are her test results from last week." She placed new papers on the table. "She placed in the eightieth percentile or higher for her age in the same skills."

I still couldn't tell what she was getting at. Her last statement sounded more suspicious than congratulatory, almost as though she was accusing me of rigging the tests.

"That's amazing," I said, grabbing the papers in disbelief. "Are you sure?" I looked up confused.

"Yes, we're sure. In fact, we even tested some of the skills again." It was quiet for a moment as I scanned the charts and graphs. When I looked up, the rest of the team was smiling.

"Mrs. Obradovic," the director took over. "Your daughter no longer qualifies for our intensive services. We're going to recommend that she still receive speech and occupational therapy in kindergarten, but she will be released from this program immediately."

I grabbed a tissue from the center of the table—the only time I have ever cried happy tears at an IEP.

The treatment plan

Our medical interventions via her medical doctors were few but effective. Among them, we restricted her diet to gluten- and casein-free foods, most of them organic and cooked at home. We also gave her digestive enzymes with every meal to help break down any proteins her body was struggling to digest.

Based on her test results, we supplemented accordingly. Mercury toxicity, confirmed by a hair test and a urine test, causes a condition that makes it very difficult for the body to transport minerals properly. In many cases, large doses of vitamin C, zinc, and calcium, for example, may be necessary to stabilize a person's mineral levels. Our doctor tailored her supplements based on her weight and individual needs to restore her levels and help facilitate the removal of mercury from her body.

We started chiropractic care. Until autism, I had always thought chiropractors were for people with bad backs. After attending a conference in May 2005, however, I learned they did so much more than that. Their philosophy, that everything in the body is affected by the ability of electric impulses to flow unobstructed through the nervous system, guided their practice of correcting the spine to make that possible. We started seeing a chiropractor weekly to correct the problems with her spine.

We also administered an antifungal to treat yeast overgrowth and added a daily dose of probiotics to replace the good flora in her digestive tract. The years and years of antibiotics had taken their toll on her ability to digest food properly. It was important to restore the proper balance of good and bad bacteria to her gut. Both helped immensely.

Emma was an immediate responder to treatment. The sensory improvements came first. By the end of the summer of 2005, she was no longer sensitive to noise. Neither the vacuum nor singing bothered her any longer, nor have they since. She also stopped flapping her hands.

The restoration of her immune system came second. Gone were the days of repeated illness and infection. In fact, with the exception of swimmer's ear, she has never had another ear infection to this day. The black circles under her eyes—they were gone, too. Emma no longer looked so sick all of the time.

Soon her skin improved. After adding prescription-strength antifungal, her eczema disappeared. The patches of it in her elbow creases and behind her knees were finally gone.

Her poops got better. Her distended and bloated belly, from her frequent constipation interspersed with bouts of diarrhea, became normal. We were able to determine that corn was a huge part of the problem. It gave her terrible diarrhea.

Her sleep got better, too. For the first time in years, Emma did not need to rock herself to sleep. The days of finding her in the glider chair or the baby swing had ended. So, too, had the night terrors.

And finally, her eyes cleared. Bright, focused, beautiful hazel beauties replaced the doped-out, glassy-looking gaze.

In addition to all of the physical improvements, developmental improvements began to show. Just as she had regressed, first physically and then developmentally, this was how she was recovering.

By winter of 2005, she showed evidence of imaginary play for the first time. Going downstairs into the basement playroom and returning with a doll and a plastic pool, she brought them to me to fill up and play with her. The moment took my breath away. Finally, at age four and a half, she was learning how to play.

Most importantly, she was learning to speak, and not just by repeating and reciting words as she had for some time, but by actually engaging in a conversation. Granted, they weren't long or detailed sentences, but they were original, conversationally appropriate thoughts she could finally express.

With each improvement I experienced a high and low. The joy and excitement of observing and participating in a new skill with her was indescribable. But even as quickly as the layers that housed her personality peeled back, I burst with impatience to tear off the rest. Every step forward only left me aching to race to the finish line faster. Gratitude and greed became my heart's constant companions as we journeyed along. They still are.

Why do elephants eat grass?

She stood quietly by the glass patio door of our new home looking outside. To my relief, there was no pool in this backyard. Instead, our new yard was filled with rectangles of freshly cut sod that had been planted along with our new landscaping. She stared at it silently for a while, something that in the past was not uncommon.

I watched her from the back, wondering what she was thinking, as always. Although she had been speaking much better for months, her speech was still delayed. I envied the ease with which other children her age could speak.

Even her younger sister, now two and a half years old, could speak better. Speech was natural for her, as it should have been. But Emma, as I suspected years before, was indeed learning English as a foreign language with nothing to go on. Her pronouns and verb tenses were still often wrong, mixed up, or absent.

"Why do elephants eat grass?" she interrupted my thoughts as she turned around to look at me curiously. I didn't think she knew I was there. Her unexpected question and behavior stopped me cold.

Did she just ask me a why question?

Before I could determine the answer, I counted the number of words she had used. Counting her words was a habit. Three- to four-word phrases were common now, but five? Five words in a row! This was a record. And not only that, she asked *why*!

I raced over to the window with an enormous smile and tears in my eyes. I held her with pure delight for a few moments before

I realized I didn't have the slightest idea why elephants eat grass. I was instantly annoyed that God would make her first question one I couldn't answer.

"I don't know, honey," I laughed as I held her tightly. "But I tell you what. We're definitely going to find out."

Always assume consciousness

I painted Emma's room the most beautiful lavender. Her white bedspread and floral accent pillows with a green gingham bed skirt and matching curtains looked serene and calm every time I entered.

From her large window, you could see directly into our side yard, where a gorgeous pear tree bloomed right in front of it every spring. Although I still didn't know her favorite color or her favorite things when I decorated it, I tried to surround her with beauty to the greatest extent possible when we moved in.

I also surrounded her with images of those who love her. On her dresser and on her desk shelves, I put pictures of her great grandmothers, grandmothers, aunts, cousins, siblings, her dad, and me. I went out of my way to make sure that everywhere she looked she would know there were people who loved her, who would always look out for her, and who would be watching over her. I even liked to believe that the images kept vigil over her in her sleep.

On one particularly beautiful spring day some time after we had gone to Disney World, I found her flipping through the Disney photo book I created for her of our trip. Like I did after all of our vacations, I had created a scrapbook for the family.

But in Emma's case, I also used photographs to help her memory. Short-term memory, especially her working memory, it appeared, had been significantly impaired. I hoped that by frequently revisiting photographs of past events, she could solidify them. I kept the little album on her nightstand for some time.

At some point, however, she put it in the top drawer. Books, crafts, Legos, stuffed animals, toy dogs, and stickers replaced most of the things I placed in the room. In a matter of only a few years, she managed to scribble in marker on her lampshade, duct tape the spindles of her desk chair, and place about a hundred animal stickers on the back of her door.

It, happily, became very much the room of a messy, creative, somewhat destructive child. Most of her family photos had been put in her closet and replaced by her collection of stuffed animals.

And so finding her relaxed on her bed quietly flipping through the small photo book from Disney World surprised me. We hadn't thought or talked about that trip for a practical reason. She was virtually nonverbal when we went.

I had no idea what she thought of Disney World, what she understood, or what she remembered. Just looking at some of the pictures made me anxious. I remembered very well how nervous and overwhelmed I was at that time.

I gently approached and asked if I could join her on the bed. She scooted over and let me look at the pictures with her. With each new page, she giggled with delight. I asked her to tell me what she was laughing about, and she did, trying to give as much detail as she could about various images.

"I loved that pool!" she claimed, pointing to the resort pool where we stayed.

"He kind of scared me," she stated, referring to the character we asked to take a photo with. You can see the uncertainty in her eyes.

I swelled with gratitude and joy realizing she actually did remember the trip. The answer to all of my fears, wondering if she was locked inside and unable to understand, or just locked inside and unable to tell me, was becoming clearer.

Emma had been in there the whole time. She just couldn't tell us. It sounds bad, but for a long time, I really wasn't sure. Did she hear me? Did she feel me? Did she know I loved her? Did she understand me? Lots of autism experts back then said no.

It's impossible to express the pain of those feelings. And it's impossible to figure out which is worse: your loved one not being able to feel you, understand you, or hear you, or your loved one not being able to tell you that they do. I imagine Alzheimer's feels the same.

The words of my mother echoed in my ears.

Always assume consciousness.

She insisted it was our responsibility to one another to assume consciousness and always behave and speak accordingly around everyone, even if we suspected they might not be able to hear us. For a long time, she reprimanded me for having any doubt that Emma was alert and well inside.

She was the one who shook me out of my sadness at what Emma couldn't do and forced me to start focusing on what she *could* do. I needed to start remembering that this was my little girl and it was my responsibility to treat her as such, she insisted. We were first and foremost a mother and a daughter, not an activist and a cause, she reminded me. My mother is a wise woman.

And so, as Emma flipped to the next photograph, the one I snapped of her red-faced and sweaty in front of the Dumbo ride, a photo I had completely forgotten taking, I held my breath ever so slightly.

I remembered the teenaged girl with autism behind us. I remembered not knowing if Emma would ever remember where we were or why it was special. I remembered all of the anxiety of trying to take a vacation, as we were just beginning biomedical interventions that summer. I cautiously asked if she remembered the ride.

"Oh, yeah!" She sat up with big eyes. "I love Dumbo!"

Which was true. Dumbo became her favorite movie over the years. She told me later that she felt like Dumbo, alone a lot of times, slow, scared, and easily confused, especially when I wasn't near. And the scene with all of the colors that looks like a hallucination? She could relate to that, too, she claimed.

"But the best part was over there," she pointed at a store in the background of the photograph. I had no idea what she was talking about.

"You took me to that candy store. I got a huge lollipop, remember?"

Holy crap, I thought, astounded. I had not, but she sure had.

The sleeping bag

When your child regresses, it is impossible not to wonder what could have been. You spend years fighting to get them back, hoping that someday they will return to the state of health and being they once had. Like a bad nightmare, you'll be able to put it all behind you someday. That's what you hope. That's what you fight for initially.

The list of things you want restored seems endless, but the basic premise is this: you want them to be healthy, happy, whole, and who they were as they came into this world. You want them to maximize their potential, be independent, and experience the most that life has to offer. It is no different from the hopes and dreams any parent has.

Among those goals is the ability to love and be loved, especially by a friend. Friends are the family we choose for ourselves, and having been blessed with the same lifelong friends for over thirty years, the thought that Emma might not ever have or make a friend devastated me in a way perhaps worse than her health.

You can be disabled in a lot of ways and still have friends. Emma was disabled in a way that prevented her from having friends. It seemed beyond cruel and unusual punishment for anyone, especially a child.

And so for years, in addition to all of the other prayers I had for her, I prayed that she would have a friend. *One friend, God.* Just one true friend is all I'm asking for. One friend that she makes on her own, whom she connects with, and who loves her back.

Emma was blessed with a lot of girls who cared about her, invited her to parties, and would even come over to play occasionally in the early years. But as she got older, the differences between them became harder to overcome, and the playdates and phone calls diminished. She needed to make a true friend. This was the ultimate sign of recovery, in my mind.

My prayer was answered in the fifth grade. She and a fellow student in her reading class became inseparable. For the entire year, they called one another, slept over at one another's houses, went to church events together, and played together without any prompting. Emma had a best friend, and I couldn't have been happier. It was magical.

One evening when she was asked to spend the night, I waited in the car while she gathered her things. For some reason, it was taking her a long time. Eventually, I grew impatient and came in to see what was wrong. Annoyed, I asked what the problem was.

"I can't find a sleeping bag," she puffed, aggravated.

"What do you mean you can't find a sleeping bag?" I puffed back at her and up the stairs. "It's in your closet."

She had received a child-sized *Little Mermaid* sleeping bag as a present several years earlier. Although she was a bit older now, it was still useful. There was no reason she couldn't take it.

I walked in her room and flipped on the light in the closet. There on the floor, among the piles of toys, books, electronics, and other items, was the absence of the sleeping bag. I could have sworn that that's where she usually kept it.

I checked her sister's room next and then the linen closet. Her brother wouldn't have it, I assumed, so I went back to her room. She was standing in the hall closet looking for something when I entered.

"I want the green one," she insisted. It was an adult sleeping bag for outdoor camping. It would work, but it was excessive. I ignored her request and kept looking.

Now thoroughly annoyed, I checked under her bed. Sure enough, pushed up against the wall near her headboard was the face of Ariel staring back at me. I grabbed it and pulled it out.

"Emma, it's right here," I said, frustrated. "Come on, let's go. I don't know why you have this smashed up under your bed like that."

She stood in front of the hall closet without moving as I walked past. I turned, perplexed and irritated.

"Come on! We have to go! You're late!"

She wouldn't budge.

"What is the problem?" I scolded.

She stood quiet for a second more before answering.

"I *hate* that sleeping bag."

Certain this was a "cool" thing and nothing more, I assured her she was not too old to have a Disney sleeping bag, and that it didn't matter anyway. She was going to her best friend's house. A best friend wouldn't care she had a *Little Mermaid* sleeping bag, but she would care if we were any later.

"That's not why I hate it," she said quietly as she stared at the ground. My patience was almost gone as I asked her to explain.

"She took her voice," she said, looking at me with a sadness I had never seen before.

"What?" I still didn't quite understand.

"She took her voice. That's what the mean witch did to her."

The enormity of what she was saying came over me. I walked to her slowly and bent down to her level.

"Oh, honey."

I didn't know how to respond for a moment. My demeanor was quiet and soft now, a complete turnaround from moments before.

"That's why you don't like *The Little Mermaid*? Because they took her voice?"

She nodded in agreement. I paused before continuing.

"And . . . you know how that feels?" I couldn't be sure this was what she meant just yet. I desperately wanted her to affirm it, but I was equally afraid she would.

"There's nothing scarier than not having your voice."

I knelt near her for a moment with my hand over my mouth symbolically speechless, feeling a combination of heartbreak and ignorant insensitivity. I was officially the worst mother in the world, I believed. Of course she would hate *The Little Mermaid*. She couldn't really speak until she was five years old, and she was aware and terrified that she couldn't the whole time.

"Come on," I grabbed her hand. "Let's go get the green one. And see this?" I held up the other. "It's going right in the garbage. You never have to see this again."

She went to the sleepover that night and had a wonderful time. At home, I threw the sleeping bag away as I said I would, along with any video, toy, or trinket that had to do with that film.

For the next year, until her best friend moved away, she used only the green sleeping bag for sleepovers. Sadly, she hasn't had to use it since then, as she hasn't had a best friend.

Gratitude and greed, I tell you, gratitude and greed.

PART III

THE RESISTANCE

Chapter 9

Activism—An Unfortunate Coincidence

By the end of summer 2005, the autism story was everywhere. Autism Speaks and Generation Rescue had launched that spring. Journalist Dan Olmsted wrote about the absence of autism among the Amish for United Press International. Robert F. Kennedy Jr. wrote a scathing article about the CDC's cover-up of the dangers of Thimerosal for *Salon* and *Rolling Stone* magazine. And journalist David Kirby went into great detail about how they did it in his book *Evidence of Harm*.

The fact that by the time I first heard the word *Thimerosal*, enough information was already out there that a book was going to print enraged me. For years, according to the story, parents worked behind the scenes to uncover what the CDC had suspected since the late 1990s: that they had made a catastrophic oversight error that led to the disabling of a generation.

When left to investigate themselves, however, they concluded they weren't guilty. Their suspicious behavior, illogical findings, and internal correspondence showed otherwise. Their behavior and their science, not the merit of vaccines, were and still are at the heart of the controversy.

But there was more to it than just mercury. In 1998, Andrew Wakefield, a gastroenterologist at the Royal Free Hospital in London, published a case study in which he and his team proposed that the live-virus measles-mumps-rubella (MMR) vaccine might be linked to autism in susceptible children. Although the paper never claimed to know whether this is the case for certain, it was retracted a decade later—the nail in the coffin used against anyone suggesting vaccines and autism are associated.

Dr. Wakefield became the poster-child of the conspiracy, his reputation and career in ruins. According to the journalist mostly responsible for his demise, and the internal investigation that subsequently ensued, Wakefield faked the entire study and orchestrated the outcome. He fiercely maintains his innocence to this day.

And although Jenny McCarthy is the most recognized celebrity face of the vaccine–autism controversy, there were other celebrities long before her that said the same. Aidan Quinn, for example, blamed vaccines, particularly the MMR, for his daughter's regression into severe nonverbal autism long before Jenny McCarthy did.

"So we had a normal child," he said in an interview in 2012, "that was walking, talking, doing everything way faster than she was supposed to. Then, after an MMR, she got a 106 fever and turned blue and woke up the next day with dark circles and not knowing who she was. And uncoordinated. And her arm lifted up. Of course the doctors are all saying, 'Oh, that's normal.'"

In 2005, however, most people still didn't know Dr. Wakefield here in the United States, certainly not by name. From what I remember, the MMR story was much more of a story in England than here. And contrary to what gets reported, hardly anyone at that time was refusing to vaccinate in the United States because of his paper. We Americans simply didn't know that much about it.

But the CDC did. And in the years leading up to 2005, they spent quite a bit of time and money investigating the two main causation theories, MMR and Thimerosal, one vaccine and one vaccine ingredient. Regarding the MMR, the CDC did epidemiological studies to make sense of Wakefield's biologically based paper.

Regarding Thimerosal, there were no studies about its safety in vaccines to go on. It had been grandfathered into use before the existence of the Food and Drug Administration, a sister agency of the Centers for Disease Control under the Department of Health and Human Services.

David Kirby's book told the whole story in detail—how a group of parents whose children regressed into autism discovered one another and the possible connection to mercury online. They were also the ones who uncovered the internal investigation of Thimerosal at the CDC.

They obtained the transcripts from Simpsonwood Retreat Center in Norcross, Georgia, on June 7 to June 8, 2000, where a secret, closed-door meeting with the world's most influential public health and vaccination experts was called by the CDC to go over the disturbing conclusions of their own study. No matter how many times the group ran the numbers, it seemed, Thimerosal appeared to be implicated in causing harm.

The lead author of the study, Dr. Thomas Verstraeten of the CDC's National Immunization Program, who immediately thereafter left to work for vaccine company Glaxo-Wellcome in Denmark, was very concerned, not only about what they had found, but also that they had gone through the trouble to find it in the first place.

According to page 31 of the transcript, he began, "It is sort of interesting that when I first came to the CDC as a NIS officer only a year ago, I didn't really know what I wanted to do, but one of the things I knew I didn't want to do was studies that had to do with toxicology or environmental health. Now it turns out that other people also thought that this study was not the right thing to do, so what I will present to you is the study nobody thought we should do."

On page 40, he continued,

> . . . we have found statistically significant relationships between the exposure and outcomes for these different exposures and outcomes. First, for two months of age, an unspecified developmental delay, which has its own specific ICD9 code. Exposure at three months of age, Tics. Exposure at six months of age, an attention deficit disorder. Exposure at one, three, and six months of age, language and speech delays which are two separate ICD9 codes. Exposures at one, three, and six months of age, the entire category of neurodevelopmental delays, which includes all of these plus a number of other disorders.

On page 42, he acknowledged they probably hadn't even identified all of the children who had been affected. "But one thing that is for sure, there is certainly an under-ascertainment of all of these because some of the children are just not old enough to be diagnosed."

And on page 161, he stated about his findings: "Personally, I have three hypotheses. My first hypothesis is it is parental bias. The children that are more likely to be vaccinated are more likely to be picked up and diagnosed. Second hypothesis, I don't know. There is a bias that I have not recognized, and nobody has yet told me about it. Third hypothesis. It's true. It's Thimerosal."

Another doctor present, Dr. Bill Weil, who represented the American Academy of Pediatrics, went even further. As we can see on page 207, he stated, "The number of dose related relationships are linear and statistically significant. You can play with this all you want. They are linear. They are statistically significant."

And yet another doctor in attendance, Dr. Brent, on page 229, made the significance of Verstraeten's findings even clearer:

> The medical/legal findings in this study, causal or not, are horrendous and therefore, it is important that the suggested

> epidemiological, pharmacokinetic, and animal studies be performed. If an allegation was made that a child's neurobehavioral findings were caused by Thimerosal containing vaccines, you could readily find junk scientists who support the claim with a 'reasonable degree of certainty'. But you would not find a scientist with any integrity who would say the reverse with the data that is available. And that is true. So we are in a bad position from the standpoint of defending any lawsuits if they were initiated and I am very concerned.

These were only a few of the statements made in the 260-page transcript that was breathtaking to read for a parent of a child with a neurodevelopmental disorder and a speech delay, in addition to a once-suspected tic (when she shook her head back and forth in her high chair). The allegations were hard to overstate.

If it had happened the way it sure looked it had, not only had the government been responsible for accidentally causing maybe the world's worst man-made medical disaster in history, they had also been allowed to investigate themselves and determine their own guilt.

The CDC group then met to discuss the findings in secret, and instead of frantically working to correct the problem and save children, they

- hemmed and hawed over whether or not the results were real or important;
- strategized about how to keep it quiet and avoid lawsuits;
- spent the next four years producing exclusively epidemiological studies designed to deny a connection, even when they acknowledged animal studies were prudent;
- finally published Verstraeten's study in 2003 after reworking the numbers and stratifying the data to claim a "neutral" outcome, the lead author literally announcing the day it was finally

presented that he was going to leave the country and work for a vaccine company;

- sent the original data sets off shore or possibly destroyed them (a crime) so that they could no longer be obtained by independent sources;
- asked the IOM to declare Thimerosal safe using a preponderance of questionable and arguably flawed population studies done in the interim;
- got an anonymous legislator (later proven to be Congressman Dick Army, R-Texas) to sneak federal protection for Eli Lilly's Thimerosal into the Homeland Security Act to protect them from any potential lawsuits (a member of the National Security Council on Homeland Security, Republican Mitch Daniels, happened to be the former Senior Vice President for Corporate Strategy and Policy at Eli Lilly and sat on their board until 2001); and

. . . did it all on the backs of vulnerable children and families.

As evidence of a possible cover-up, one attendee of Simpsonwood, Dr. Bill Egan of the FDA's Center for Biologics Evaluation and Research, testified under oath to Congress only a month later, on July 18, 2000, that there was no credible evidence of any link between Thimerosal and neurodevelopmental disorders, even though he had just spent two days behind closed doors going over the very study that showed there was.

That certainly seemed like fraud to us, but that is not a small accusation, and all of us knew it. How fierce, ruthless, and orchestrated the defense would be, however, I'm not so sure any of us knew.

An unfortunate coincidence

David Kirby made his rounds in the media defending his work. He is an award-winning investigative journalist and author who had written for the *New York Times*. His most recent book, *Death at SeaWorld*, played a role in SeaWorld's decision to stop breeding killer whales in captivity.

Given that this was prior to the age we now live in, where online commenting is a blood sport, and journalists with controversial findings about vaccines were still allowed to go on television (in 2010 the Obama administration asked for media censorship), he made many appearances.

The world was interested in what he had to say, for the Institute of Medicine in May 2004, at the request of the CDC in Task Order 74 (a one-page memo that defines the study they are asking the IOM to do that they have refused to release to the public), had supposedly closed the door on this topic.

Although in 2001 the IOM concluded that the theories that mercury in vaccines and the MMR vaccine could cause autism had merit and were biologically plausible, within three years, they flipped their position 180 degrees. Not only weren't the theories any longer plausible, they claimed, they went so far as to say neither topic ever needed to be studied again. David's book provided evidence of possible corruption being the reason for these developments.

And so he appeared on *Meet the Press* on August 7, 2005, with the late Tim Russert. Tim was one of the most trusted personalities in television news at the time. All of us looked forward to his show with excitement. If anyone would give David a fair chance, it was Tim.

Opposite David, to counter his claims, was Dr. Harvey Feinberg. He considered what David said carefully and then responded. While I didn't like what he said and strongly disagreed, the conversation between them remained very professional. In the end, however, there was no common ground between them.

The discussion reminded me a lot of the articles I was reading at that time, balanced in coverage, but concluding Thimerosal was safe. Dr. Feinberg predictably refuted the evidence of a link between

Thimerosal and autism and defended the actions of the CDC and other agencies in their exoneration of it.

"It's an unfortunate coincidence," I heard someone once say. That parents were noticing their children's autism at the time of their vaccinations was an unfortunate coincidence. It was essentially the same message here.

Autism, and all that surrounded its onset, its symptoms, its recovery, its explosion, its controversy, their findings, their behavior, and their correspondence, was a coincidence. It was almost worse than being accused of not loving Emma enough.

According to organized medicine, it seemed clear: I was not only cold, heartless, and genetically flawed—the three most accepted causation theories of autism in history—I might also be crazy. Although, to be fair, doctors never used those words, they did repeatedly imply that I couldn't trust my own reality. They insisted that I was wrong when I claimed Emma wasn't born with autism, that she truly had regressed before my eyes, and that with treatment, she was getting better.

And hell if they weren't set on making the world believe it no matter what it took. Ten years later, they have done exactly that.

An evening for autism

Within a year of David Kirby's book, I became an outspoken critic of the CDC and their claims about Thimerosal safety. I frequently commented on stories and threads. I wrote essays about our journey. I flew to Washington, DC, to attend a rally with friends I made online. I met with my senator and representatives, and I protested in front of the National Institutes of Health.

And as Emma improved, I started to think about how I could give back. Treating her had been expensive. We spent thousands on medical, physical, speech, academic, and occupational therapies and interventions, not including conferences and travel. There was no way a lot of people would be able to afford that.

So in late 2006, I decided to throw a benefit and asked David Kirby to be the guest speaker. I invited everyone I knew, hired a DJ and a professional photographer, and organized a silent auction. Almost 500 people attended it in February 2007. We raised thousands of dollars.

That night I spoke along with David. Many people, including him, complimented my speech, where I made an analogy that no one else had at that point. Our children were metaphorically on fire, I said, and while some people were standing around debating whether or not there was a fire, whether smoke was associated, and what, if anything, should be done about it, there were those of us who had gotten the hell out of the house and were grabbing anything we could to put it out.

When we were somewhat successful in our attempt, however, we were attacked for the kind of water we had chosen. In their view, toilet water was not a great way to put out a fire, nor had it ever been studied for effectiveness. In fact, these critics argued, they still weren't even sure there was a fire to begin with.

I got good laughs, but nothing about that analogy was funny. It is exactly what has happened to parents trying to help their children with autism. We only think our children are on fire, they claim. They have the symptoms of being burned, yes, and they have been exposed to fire, yes, but they actually haven't been burned. Furthermore, doing anything to eliminate the fire and treat their burns is unnecessary and dangerous.

No one knows anything . . .

The day after the fundraiser, I organized a speaking engagement for David at the school where I taught. Not long before then, I had been invited by one of my administrators to present on autism to the faculty at an in-service day. He asked me at approximately four o'clock in the afternoon on a Thursday to present the following morning.

"No one knows anything about autism," he insisted, convincing me to take the opportunity. "It's always been so rare. You're in a unique position to educate the staff about this condition that's suddenly showing up in our classrooms."

All of that was true. It was rare. None of us, including him, had ever known anyone with the condition. And none of the teachers outside of the special education department had the slightest clue how to teach a student diagnosed with it.

But that included me, I told him. My daughter was only six years old. Anything we knew about educating a child with autism was coming from the elementary schools, because prior to that, we hadn't needed to know. It was right around 2006 or 2007 that the epidemic started hitting the high schools. It was that year our school began an autism program for the first time.

I thought about it for maybe an hour before agreeing to do it. I knew I wouldn't have near enough time to do a thorough job on the subject, but at least I could educate everyone about the controversy.

Perhaps I could just get everyone thinking about why we needed to learn how to teach these students all of a sudden. Where had they been? Why did we now need an autism program when for the entire history of the school it had never been necessary?

But even that conversation scared me. I was smart enough to know that talking about the epidemic, calling it that, and God forbid, bringing up CDC corruption and vaccines as a cause were a huge risk.

I got along wonderfully with all of my colleagues. They liked me, and I liked them. I had a great reputation as a professional. Talking about this could change that forever. I was scared out of my mind.

I was equally afraid not to, however. Many of my teacher friends were young people getting married and having babies. *Two colleagues I was close with went on to have affected children within five years.*

This was serious stuff. They needed to understand the experience of tens of thousands of parents across the globe right now, including me. At the least, they needed to be aware of the other side of the story. I decided it was more important to plant a seed than be well liked.

As I expected, I got mixed reviews. People who knew me well were supportive and complimentary. People who thought I was off base kept it to themselves, except for one. A colleague I had been close with emailed a rebuttal to the staff. He let everyone know that he thought I was misguided. It hurt, but it wasn't unexpected.

And so David Kirby being in town to back me up was a welcome event in my mind. If they didn't believe me, that was okay. Maybe a serious journalist with a book might be more effective.

On the Sunday after the fundraiser, about fifty people showed up to hear him speak, many of them the teachers who supported me. The colleague who didn't agree, unfortunately, was not one of them.

The age of autism advocacy

The year 2007 proved to be an important one for the controversy. Until that year, the words "vaccines and autism" had not been said together on television outside of David Kirby's interviews. (Last year, in 2015, it was hard not to hear them, especially when the measles outbreak took place.)

To my recollection, the first person to say them on a mainstream television show was Jenny McCarthy, which is a lot of the reason she receives so much of the disdain for the link. But Holly Robinson Pete once shared the stage with Jenny McCarthy. And most people don't remember that Katie Wright, the daughter of the founders of Autism Speaks, did, too.

They had been invited to *The Oprah Winfrey Show* to share their stories as mothers of affected children. Even though all three of them agreed vaccines had played a role in their children's regression, and they all repeatedly stated they were not anti-vaccine, they were immediately and forever after treated as such.

Jenny's exact words were "What number will it take for people to start listening to what the mothers of children with autism have been saying for years, which is 'We vaccinated our baby and something happened'?"

It was a thoughtful and honest question. She didn't say, "Don't vaccinate!"

She didn't say, "All vaccines are bad!"

In fact, on every single appearance she made thereafter, she reiterated that she wasn't against vaccination. She was against bad policy, sketchy science, and the most aggressive, one-size-fits-all, for-profit, vaccination schedule in the world that has never once been tested for safety in the real-world way in which it is administered (giving four or five vaccines from different manufacturers at once while on antibiotics and/or acetaminophen, for example).

But it didn't matter. Once the other side decides what they want the world to remember you by on this issue, they don't let up until they get it. The definition of being anti-vaccine has been made very clear. If you're not all for, you are all against. There is no room for middle ground, and even the implication that there's cause for a concern is considered irresponsible and dangerous.

I remember watching her say the words in awe. The audience was full of mothers like me, and a few of them whom I had gotten to know well online happened to be there. I watched their faces as Jenny spoke, most of them becoming teary-eyed with relief. Finally, someone had articulated our experience. And finally, someone was listening.

The NAA conference

Jenny was a speaker at the National Autism Association conference in Atlanta that November. For months, she made the talk-show rounds and quickly became a lightning rod for the controversy. Like me, she claimed she had made a deal with God that if He gave the ability to heal her child, she would dedicate her life to helping other families do the same.

I had made the same deal when Emma's younger sister became ill with an ear infection in the exact same month as Emma's first. I fell to my knees that night, crying and begging that if God would spare me that child, I would help affected children and families for the rest of my life. He made good on his end of the deal, and I am trying to make good on mine.

So I was happy to fly to Atlanta to see Jenny speak. Admittedly, I was also anxious to meet some more of my new friends in person. This was my fourth conference in three years, and by then, conferences were not only a tremendous source of inspiration and information, they also offered me a lifeline of emotional support.

The parents at these conferences "got it." I didn't have to explain anything to them. I didn't have to choose my words wisely, wondering if they were judging me or questioning my stability. I could discuss autism all day, every day, and no one cared. In fact, that's all they wanted to talk about, too.

I could bring up anything from poop problems to eczema to brands of supplements, and they knew exactly what I meant. I could go from discussing a sophisticated scientific study in one breath to brainstorming meaningful legislation for our kids in the next.

I could also spontaneously burst into tears for any reason, and someone would reach over and give me a hug without question, often someone I didn't know. And I could spend three days in a beautiful hotel with other like-minded adults, having adult conversations, not thinking about work, not running errands or doing dishes, and physically removing myself from the stress that was now my home life.

That kind of connection was indescribable. It was also addictive. I was bonded with people from around the country I had just met in a way that was stronger than many of my lifelong relationships. These people understood me. They spoke my language. And many of them inspired me. They were *smart.* They were well connected. And they were determined to make a difference. I was like a moth drawn to a flame when it came to conferences, especially when it became clear that the people I admired so much felt the same way about me.

But I instinctively felt nervous about it, too. Mike didn't come with me to most of the conferences. I would tell myself it was for practical reasons, as it was no doubt very difficult for both of us to go. The expense, the time off work, and the child-care arrangements certainly did make it a challenge.

But it was more than that. Mike and I didn't connect over autism. We actually disconnected over it. He had no desire to leap into the virtual world and share his life or pain. He is an extremely private person. He would never do such a thing.

And so he didn't know these people I now considered close friends by more than their names. He tried to seem interested, but it was obvious he was not. I sensed that he tolerated my endless conversations about them and what we did, but I could also sense that he resented it.

And whether I wanted to admit it or not, I knew I was growing resentful of him, too. His "support"—never giving me a hard time about going to the conferences or spending so much time online—felt more like ambivalence after a while.

Plenty of fathers came to these conferences. Plenty of them were mad as hell, starting organizations, blogging, meeting with legislators, and speaking out. Plenty of them took detailed notes on complicated medical issues and went out of their way to learn as much as they could to help their child.

I interpreted Mike's lack of doing the same as not caring as much about Emma as I did. I certainly didn't verbalize it that way, but I felt it. And that is the exact same dangerous feeling any mother has when her child is threatened or rejected.

Now instead of just feeling resentful, angry, and afraid of the medical community, I was also quietly burning with resentment, anger, and fear toward my husband. I worried deeply that autism would eventually tear us apart, even though I was always able to talk myself out of it. And because of this, selfishly perhaps, I kept involving myself in the controversy and going to the conferences anyway. I had to.

For truthfully, I was primarily going to these conferences to continue helping Emma. By the fall of 2007, at the start of first grade, two years after beginning treatment, even though so many issues, such as her repeated illnesses, her sensory problems, her eye contact, her speech, and her gut, had either completely resolved or improved by then, her learning disabilities and social deficits had not.

Emma still struggled immensely with reading comprehension and abstract thought. Academically and socially, she was way behind. At age seven, she had the interests of a four- or five-year-old. Even to this day, she consistently remains about three to five years younger emotionally than her peers. Her mental and chronological ages are not the same.

These were the next areas of disability that I needed to focus on intensely, and the main reason why I had flown to Atlanta. Unexpectedly, the years would prove they would be the hardest area of her autism to overcome. Emma still struggles with them today.

On one of the conference days, I found myself in the giant ballroom almost alone. I sat down to wait for the next speaker and look through my notes when, behind me, Dan Olmsted and Mark Blaxill appeared. Dan was the journalist who had written the series *Age of Autism* for UPI. Mark was the father of an affected child, and was one of the original parents instrumental in bringing CDC corruption to light, a Harvard- and Princeton-educated man, and one of the smartest people I had ever met.

Together, they told me, they were starting a new blog that would go live any day. The current blog, *The Rescue Post*, would be taken over by *Age of Autism. The Rescue Post* had been launched approximately the year before as an alternative to the chat rooms. J. B. Handley, the father and founder of Generation Rescue, had created it. Dan's series would become the name of the new blog. It would be the first daily web newspaper about the autism epidemic.

I was thrilled. In the year prior, I had come to know Dan and Mark and their work well. I admired them immensely, and I was excited for what they could do with this new platform. Rumor had it that all of the organizations that viewed autism medically, such as Generation Rescue, National Autism Association, and Talk About Curing Autism, were organizing during the conference to discuss becoming one organization, the antithesis of Autism Speaks.

Autism Speaks had quickly identified itself mostly as a genetically oriented organization. It was offering parents nothing in terms of treatment or support of any kind. These other organizations, all founded with the money of parents of affected children, not the millions of the founder of Home Depot, Bernie Marcus, were doing remarkable things on a shoestring budget.

They had journey guides, recipe books, mentoring programs, IEP assistance, support groups, research projects, treatment grants, emergency hotlines, and so much more. Together, the hope was, they could be the alternative autism group, a true force to be reckoned with when it came to funding.

In 2006, the first federal legislation regarding autism had come down the pike. The Combating Autism Act had been passed, not without controversy, and now millions of dollars were available for those scientists and organizations that could prove they could put it to use. Scientists and researchers began competing for grants to research their causation paradigms, genetic or environmental.

Our small organizations that believed in the environmental paradigm of autism causation couldn't compete with the genetically leaning Autism Speaks when it came to securing grants, but a new, combined organization might. It was imperative we try.

Unfortunately, for reasons unknown to me, the merger never took place. I often wonder what would have happened if it had. But on that day, in that ballroom, it was still a real possibility. And on that day, in that ballroom, Dan and Mark asked me to join their blog as a contributing editor. I gladly and humbly accepted.

Chapter 10

Anger—A Vaccine for Autism, or Something Like It

Although it wasn't slated as the keynote address, it very well could have been. The National Autism Association had gotten the National Institutes of Health to come to their annual conference, this year in Atlanta, Georgia. Dr. Tom Insel, the appointed leader of the new task force created by the Combating Autism Act, the Interagency Autism Coordinating Committee (IACC), was coming to speak.

It was a big deal. Until then, November 2007, autism conferences were frequently criticized for not being scientifically based. Accusations of selling hope and snake oil were common and would only get worse.

Having the head of IACC present not only opened the door for parents to ask questions and feel heard, it also legitimized the conference. Significantly, I felt, it was also one of the first conferences where Jenny McCarthy was speaking.

And so I waited in the ballroom patiently with other parents making sure to get a seat. It was the same ballroom where Dan Olmsted and Mark Blaxill had just asked me to join the *Age of Autism* team, only this time, I sat almost all the way to the left of the stage toward the back.

A couple of friends of mine, Kevin and Becky, both activists and parents of affected children, joined me. We made small talk, discussed other presentations, and made each other laugh. Their friendships, as well as the many others I have gained through autism advocacy, have been some of the most important I've ever had.

I couldn't wait to hear what Dr. Insel had to say. For two years, I felt like I had something to prove to explain why we thought autism was environmentally caused and why we were pursuing the treatments we were. Dr. Insel was as mainstream and respected as anyone could be. He was from the National Institutes of Health, for crying out loud. If he confirmed what we knew, that our children were physically ill, not mentally ill, it would be a game changer.

Another doctor and he stood on the stage together. For a while their presentation felt disappointing, as they weren't offering us any new or interesting insights, and I found myself distracted by my friend's sarcastic and humorous comments. It was during one of his jokes that I happened to look up and see these words across the two gigantic screens behind the speakers:

A VACCINE FOR AUTISM

My eyes bulged and my mouth dropped. I gasped, laughing ever so slightly in shock, and nudged my friend while pointing, wide-eyed.

"Look!" I whispered in utter and complete shock, bumping his arm. "Look!"

He made the same face and then looked at me. It was impossible to process the significance of what those words meant, but our expressions said it all. Either Dr. Insel had no idea who his audience was and how insanely insensitive that was to suggest, or he didn't care.

The room slowly started buzzing, a ripple of heads turning, pointing, and starting sidebar conversations moving across the chairs in a wave. Imagine the NIH hosting a conference on lung cancer and offering a cigarette as prevention, and you may have some idea how the energy shifted.

Although it was hard, I tried to concentrate. I always give people the benefit of the doubt, and I began to think maybe there was something to this. Perhaps it meant they identified a virus or bacteria in our children that could be prevented. While I believed it wouldn't have been there in the first place without vaccine injury, I was encouraged that they appeared to be investigating the condition medically.

"And that's why some day, we hope," Dr. Insel continued sincerely, "We'll have a vaccine for autism, or something like it."

I shook my head, stunned. Parents of severely affected children looked around as if to say, "Can you believe this? Is this guy for real?"

I worried someone would get up and confront him, but nothing like that happened. In fact, no one really moved.

A few minutes later, Jenny entered the ballroom and sat on the left side of the room close to where we sat. The words had not been removed from the screen yet, just hanging there over our heads, staring back at hundreds of parents of children who had regressed into autism within hours or weeks of receiving the vaccines; parents who had flown from around the country to try to help their children by coming to this conference.

They were also taxpayers, the ones funding the IACC, and they had a financial interest in the direction that money was going and who was in charge of it. Dr. Insel was that guy. *This* is what he intended—"a vaccine for autism." It wasn't good.

When the presentation ended, the audience was given a chance to ask questions. A microphone was placed in one of the aisles, and a long line of people formed behind it. Almost every question and comment revolved around the insensitivity and ignorance of that comment to this audience.

Most importantly, the energy of not only the room, but also the movement felt different to me from that moment on. I believe until then, parents felt frustrated and skeptical, yet hopeful. From that moment forward, including up to this day, however, there was only one emotion I could truly sense among my peers, and shortly thereafter, from those on the receiving end of it as well.

Anger.

Hannah Poling

A few months later, on March 7, 2008, something incredible happened. One of the children among the 5,000 that had been grouped together in what was called an omnibus proceeding to be heard by the "vaccine court" of the Court of Federal Claims to determine whether autism had been caused by vaccines had quietly been pulled and awarded on the side.

Her parents, Jon and Terry Poling, a neurologist and nurse/lawyer respectively, had decided to come forward publicly with their story and host a press conference with the news. It was an extraordinary display of courage.

Dr. and Mrs. Poling described in detail how their daughter received nine vaccinations in one visit and went on to have a seizure later that day. Hannah, they claimed, was never the same. Eventually, she was diagnosed with severe autism, and they sued for damages in the federal vaccine compensation program where they received a multimillion-dollar settlement.

Unbeknownst to most Americans, Congress passed legislation in the mid-1980s to grant the pharmaceutical industry that created childhood vaccines—as well as the doctors and medical practitioners who administered them—liability protection from being held accountable for specific harm caused by protected vaccines (as outlined in the Vaccine Injury Table of the 1986 National Childhood Vaccine Injury Act).

As a result, the National Vaccine Injury Compensation Program (known as the VICP) was created under the National Childhood Vaccine Injury Act of 1986. From that point forward, rather than being able to directly sue the pharmaceutical companies or their doctors for damages, parents who suspected a vaccine injury in their child would have to sue the United States government in a claims court nicknamed "Vaccine Court." (A civil suit may be filed in a state or federal court without first filing a petition in the VICP if requesting damages of $1,000 or less.)

Special masters appointed by the government would rule. Together, they would determine the allowable evidence and what merit it had. As long as the plaintiff could demonstrate reasonable causation, they were instructed to compensate the injured party.

"Fifty percent and a feather," a lawyer once told me. That was supposed to be all you needed to win. Interestingly, if you did win, however, you would essentially end up paying yourself. Vaccines carry a small excise tax that funds the compensation court. To date, over three billion dollars has been paid out from money collected through other consumers.

It's hard not to argue in favor of the court in some respects. Certainly the private sector had a point. If they were going to be asked by the government to create a product recommended by the government for children, and often mandated by state law, they shouldn't be responsible for carrying the weight of liability alone.

But, as always, the devil is in the details.

To begin, it opened the floodgates for childhood vaccine development. Without the worry of liability, pharmaceutical companies had every incentive to create as many childhood vaccines as possible, as quickly as possible. It is not a coincidence, I believe, that within fifteen years of this legislation, we went from three recommended vaccines given multiple times each (that addressed seven different diseases, the MMR, the DTaP, and polio) for American children to seven total vaccines also given multiple times each (adding vaccines to address hepatitis B, Hib, rotavirus, and varicella)—more than double what they had ever received before. It is not a coincidence, I believe, that the list of recommended childhood vaccines has continued to grow in the last fifteen years and now recommends seventy vaccine doses for an American child from birth through age eighteen.

But worst of all, this legislation opened the floodgates for lobbying. Not only could the industry avoid liability, it could also lobby to mandate their product's use. For the first time where vaccines were concerned, a child's best interest could be in direct conflict with the best interest of a pharmaceutical company's bottom line, without any way to hold the pharmaceutical company accountable.

Also troubling is the fact that there is a revolving door between our regulatory bodies and our pharmaceutical industry that many Americans, specifically parents, are extremely concerned about. Dr. Julie Gerberding, for example, head of the CDC during the George W. Bush administration, left her post upon its termination to be president of Merck's vaccine division after the legally required one year and one day. The very person responsible for ensuring vaccine uptake and vaccine safety went to work for a vaccine company after her tenure. It's suspicious at best.

Equally troublesome is the fact that there are often tremendous conflicts of interest among members of the committee responsible for adding new vaccines to the childhood recommended schedule (known as the Advisory Committee on Immunization Practices, or ACIP).

Believe it or not, some members of the ACIP were even vaccine developers themselves. Dr. Paul Offit is an example. He is the creator of a rotavirus vaccine that was eventually granted liability protection under the Vaccine Injury Compensation Program (VICP) in 1998. But he was also a member of the ACIP, which was determining whether or not to add it to the vaccine schedule, during that time.

It is important to note he abstained from the ACIP vote due to his conflict; however, it perfectly illustrates the potential for problems. Many of the remaining voting members in that instance received consulting fees, educational grants, travel expenses, and/or owned stock in a pharmaceutical company their vote would affect, although they had disclosed this on waiver forms.

And finally, there is another concern. Legislation also passed in the 1980s, known as the Bayh-Dole Act, allows for something called a public–private partnership. In essence, researchers and developers in the public sector, such as those working at the National Institutes of Health, are now legally allowed to license their products to the private sector for profit.

The human papilloma virus vaccine, commonly known as Gardasil, came to the market in this very way. Its technology was developed at the National Cancer Institute under the NIH and was licensed to Merck, which created Gardasil. The NIH, a sister agency of the CDC and FDA, operating under the Department of Health and Human Services, receives a royalty from every vaccine sold.

This means that the DHHS is technically the same entity that created the vaccine, profits from the vaccine, determines its safety, and is the defendant in the court that determines if a consumer is injured. This is an unprecedented, and arguably outrageous, situation.

Dan Olmsted and Mark Blaxill wrote a stunning explanation of how it happened and its implications first in a series for their blog *Age of Autism* and later as a chapter in the book *Vaccine Epidemic,* called "A License to Kill."

The DHHS can kill a consumer with their product, make money while doing it, participate in the investigation, and largely determine their own liability. And once again, the very person in charge of the CDC when Gardasil was added to the schedule, Dr. Julie Gerberding, now works for the company that makes it.

Intentional or not, the VICP legislation and childhood recommended schedule provided the pharmaceutical industry with a never-ending stream of consumers through children. Getting a new vaccine added to the recommended schedule meant billions of dollars in revenue for them. It still does.

And so the addition of four new vaccines to the recommended schedule shortly after liability protection took effect was not surprising. As a result, for the first time, we were not only vaccinating on the first day of birth, we were also routinely vaccinating babies with more than one injection at once, such as the nine given to Hannah in one day, something that still hasn't been tested for safety.

It is exactly when we started this practice in the early 1990s that the explosion in the documented cases of autism and other neurodevelopmental disorders began. It is also exactly when the cracks in the program's design first began to show. Without safeguarding liability protection from private industry influence, we provided no incentive for industry restraint.

Without the addition of an independent oversight agency for vaccine safety science, one without ties to the pharmaceutical industry and outside of the Department of Health and Human Services, we provided no unbiased checks and balances.

The CDC suddenly became the agency both responsible for increasing vaccine uptake and for identifying and admitting vaccine injury, the equivalent of serving two masters. I'm confident this is because when the CDC was created, no one ever suspected the very agency responsible for controlling disease outbreak could someday be the same agency that caused one.

Investigators from an independent oversight agency might have stopped the Thimerosal controversy in its tracks, but we will never know. Perhaps they would have realized that the two new vaccines, coming from different pharmaceutical companies, both contained the mercury-based preservative in large amounts. Perhaps they would have done the math and discovered that their addition to the schedule not only moved the exposure to Thimerosal up to the day of birth, but also nearly tripled the amount a child could be exposed to.

But such an oversight organization didn't exist, so it couldn't. And children were suddenly exposed to up to three times the amount of mercury they ever had been exposed to before, at an earlier age than ever. And by the mid-1990s, children were showing the signs and symptoms of neurological problems that might be explained by mercury exposure in alarming numbers, which in part prompted the government's investigation.

Although the CDC acknowledges they tripled the amount without realizing it, they maintain to this day that nothing happened as a result, claiming that any and all correlating neurological injuries are nothing more than another unfortunate coincidence. They have even presented evidence that their oversight error was a blessing in disguise. Thimerosal, some of their science shows, appears to prevent autism.

Interestingly, in my own life, I can't accidentally triple my exposure to anything toxic without consequence. If I drink three glasses of wine versus one, there's a big difference. If I smoke three packs of cigarettes versus one, my risk of cancer skyrockets. If I take three times the amount of medication I'm prescribed, I can die.

In fact, I can't really think of anything in life, toxic in its natural state, that we can triple our exposure to without consequence. The government, however, has found it. Thimerosal in vaccines, they tell us, is the exception. And not only that, it's good for us, too.

Liability-free? Vaccine-free

The reaction of parents to the legislation and to the aggressive, liability-free, and pharmaceutically friendly vaccine schedule exclusively employed in the United States was predictable. It was only logical it would happen. People would stop vaccinating.

With 1 in 68 children affected by autism, 1 in 8 children in special education, and over 50 percent of children with a chronic disease as of today, parents would have no choice but to question what was happening. With tens of thousands of parents blaming vaccines, it was only natural that the friends, family, neighbors, and colleagues of affected families would take heed.

By 2015, they had. In many states, particularly those with philosophical exemptions, the vaccine compliance rate dropped. Religious exemptions in other states were also going up. Although most parents did not want to forego vaccination completely, they wanted to have more of a say regarding which vaccines their children would receive. They knew they didn't live in a cesspool of disease in the 1980s, and they weren't buying that their children would either if they didn't give them all forty-nine recommended doses before kindergarten.

But that made medical leadership angry. They didn't like being questioned by parents. And even though CDC-funded studies were identifying parents who were unlikely to vaccinate as highly educated parents, they felt little problem admonishing these parents' stupidity. Some doctors even went so far as to expel them from their practice, or politely suggest they were no longer a good fit, like our doctors had with us. Who were these parents to tell these doctors how to do their job? Had they gone to medical school?

Sometimes they had. In most cases, they were either the parents of a child who had regressed into autism trying to protect a younger sibling from the same fate, hardly a radical desire, or they were people who knew the parents of children with developmental delays warning them to educate themselves about vaccines, toxins, antibiotics, and other medications before they did anything. Contrary to the popular "anti-vaccine" caricature, these were not crazy people.

They also had a legitimate unanswered question. How was it that the only thing the medical community knew for sure about autism and the other disorders popping up and growing exponentially was that vaccines had nothing to do with them? It was suspicious at best.

And so the trust began to dwindle, and anger began to stew. Explanations, even though false, spread like wildfire. Jenny McCarthy! Tin-foil hat parents! Andrew Wakefield! These were the culprits, supposedly.

Those of us on the inside knew that absolutely wasn't true. Educated parents who had followed their doctor's orders to a T and ended up with a brain-damaged child anyway simply didn't trust the CDC, the medical leadership, or the pharmaceutical industry with their children's health any longer.

More vaccines, more antibiotics, and more medicine were clearly not correlated with better health. Throughout the last few decades, the more of each was administered, the more chronic illness and disability children had.

And to deny the power of the pharmaceutical industry, the most powerful lobby in Congress, was insane. Perhaps this wasn't in my child's best interest after all, parents realized, looking at the recommended chart and the legislation and conflicts of interest that made their children a cash cow. They began to opt out.

The response to that, however, was also predictable. Rather than look internally for reasons they had lost parents' trust, medical leadership doubled down on their defense. They no longer care if you trust them. You're going to do what they say regardless.

Legislation across the country appeared in 2015 with one main agenda: get rid of choice. No parent or citizen shall have the right to opt out of the vaccine program and participate in society, they say. We either do what they say on time every time, or we lose the right to be in public.

No exemptions. No exceptions. For none of us lay people are qualified to question them or their science. And they are done messing around. Some states have even gone so far as to threaten parents with taking away their children or with jail time.

California was perhaps the greatest example. Until 2015, its residents had the right to a philosophical exemption. After the outbreak of measles that affected fewer than 200 people, however, all of whom recovered and went on to have lifelong immunity, a war against exemptions began. It was the perfect backdrop, and, as I later learned right before testifying to an Illinois Senate committee, the perfect timing organized medicine had been waiting for.

Their plan was simple. Blame bad parents, bad doctors, and bad celebrities for the outbreak and putting people at risk. Shame parents of brain-damaged kids who were exempting their other children out of precaution. Present the doctors and the medical community as the real victims of this problem. Scare the crap out of everyone by suggesting that they are all going to die because of these "anti-vaccine" monsters.

And all the while, the media gladly assisted, *Time* magazine even going so far as to suggest making a public registry of noncompliant families available on the web with their addresses.

By the end of the summer, however, it had worked. Vaccine exemptions in California were gone. Pharmaceutical lobbyists rejoiced in the aisles of the government building where the vote took place, thrilled to have taken away parental rights, convinced they had protected lives by doing so.

The same happened in many other states, mostly blue ones, and is still happening today. Democrats tend to favor vaccine mandates more than Republicans. Regardless, both parties refuse to see what the real issue is.

No matter how hard you try, you can't legislate trust. Mark my words, especially as the medical industrial complex is poised to tie vaccine mandates to everyone's health coverage and welfare benefits in the future, and as it has already begun to attempt it with military personnel, this fight has only just begun.

But back in 2008, mandates and legislation, and the anger that would come with both, were just beginning to bubble up. The Polings coming forward with their story, how and why Hannah had been the victim of brain damage, and how and why their case had been secretly pulled and awarded on the side, put more fuel on the fire. Hannah was fine. Hannah got vaccinated. Hannah got autism. And Hannah got awarded for it. People were pissed.

I was one of them, but not because Hannah got compensated. I was pissed because I had never even heard of the vaccine court when Emma regressed. I had no idea such a thing existed, let alone that there was a statute of limitations on the time you could take to file a claim. By 2008, our time had run out.

Even if it were ever proven that Emma's doctors and the vaccines they gave her had in any way hurt her, she would never see a dime.

Not one doctor had warned me about the potential side effects I should look for, such as rashes, fevers, encephalopathy, high-pitched screaming, seizures, or eczema. Not one doctor had adhered to the contraindications or precautions to vaccinating, such as moderate or severe acute illness with or without fever (like, say, an ear infection?). Not one doctor had reported her rash or any of her symptoms to the Vaccine Adverse Event Reporting System, a national vaccine safety surveillance created under the 1986 National Childhood Vaccine Injury Act. Not one doctor had told me about my rights or my lack of them.

The Polings had an advantage, I felt. He was a neurologist. She was a nurse and a lawyer, hardly tin-foil-hat–wearing conspiracy theorists. They knew people. They knew what to ask. And they knew what tests to run. It was determined Hannah had an underlying mitochondrial disorder that made her vulnerable to vaccine injury.

I would have never known to test for something like that, and neither would most parents. According to the careful wording of the ruling, she was the exception, the one child of the 5,000 in the United States whose parents were reporting a similar problem post-vaccination.

Apparently, they explained, she had an underlying disorder that was exacerbated by vaccination, which resulted in the features of autism, but she didn't actually have autism, and the vaccinations didn't cause it. It was the equivalent of claiming you have an underlying metabolic disorder that was exacerbated by food resulting in the features of fat, but that you aren't actually fat, and food had nothing to do with it.

Furthermore, and more importantly, the government couldn't determine whether her mitochondrial problem was the cause of or the result of her vaccination reaction. Although they implied she had some genetic abnormality from birth, her parents insisted that was not true, and this was part of the reason they came forward. And mercury is a known mitochondrial disruptor. In fact, more than 20 percent of children with autism present with some kind of mitochondrial problem.

The truth is, Hannah Poling was no different from so many of our children, no matter how hard the government wanted to make it otherwise. Still, she remains the exception in the eyes of the medical community, the rare anomaly that unfortunately got hurt.

Even if the claim were true, we argued, that she had an underlying condition making her vulnerable to vaccine damage, why is nothing being done to identify kids like her before vaccinating them? How will we ever know who is vulnerable to vaccination injury if we don't?

What discovery will discover

In the years since, those who defend the bloated vaccine schedule, the mandates, and the one-size-fits-all program for everyone also defend the vaccine compensation program. They also claim that no one is prohibited from taking a case that was not awarded by the Vaccine Injury Compensation Program and going on their own afterward to a traditional court. That is true. Anyone claiming vaccine injury may do so.

What they won't tell you, however, is that it usually takes years in the federal compensation court before you get a ruling. They won't tell you that the government has been very unreliable, and arguably defiant, about making sure plaintiffs' lawyers receive payment, shrinking the pool of those willing to take on these cases so that it is by now very, very small.

They won't tell you that eighty-three cases have been compensated for vaccine injury that involve autism, but all of them were awarded in cases where the plaintiffs did not use the word "autism" in their claim.

They also won't tell you the cost involved, nor do they consider that these families are simultaneously dealing with a brain-damaged child, one who often needs round-the-clock care and services. After already spending thousands of dollars and hours on their case in federal court for years, they now have to decide how much more money and time they can afford on their own to sue the entire medical industrial complex.

One side has a sick, brain-damaged child to take care of on their own. One side has all of the power, influence, and money to make that case drag on a lifetime if they choose (the same side that funds, executes, and reports on all of the evidence that would be brought into court to be used against them anyway).

Is it really any surprise very few families decide to do this?

"Green Our Vaccines"

June 4, 2008 was a scorching day in Washington, DC. The air was thick and humid. That morning in the dim sun, we stood on the National Mall near the Washington monument, thousands of us gathered to march. I was wearing my brightly colored lime-green shirt with the words "Green Our Vaccines" across the front, helping to get the other protesters organized.

By most estimates, there were approximately 8,000 people who came. I had hoped for a larger turnout, but of all of the rallies in DC I had been to by that point, this by far was the biggest. Plus, with the celebrity presence of Jenny McCarthy and Jim Carrey, who along with a few autism organizations were responsible for the rally, I knew it would get a lot of media attention. It was enough.

We walked the streets of the capital, weaving in and out of various sectors, and eventually came to rest on the huge lawn behind the Capitol Building. There we waited anxiously to hear from the speakers on the stage, among them Jenny, Jim, Dr. Boyd Haley, and Robert F. Kennedy, Jr. Music played, and everyone gathered closely with their posters and children to hear what they had to say. Behind us was a sea of cameras, microphones, and reporters doing the same.

It should have been an inspiring experience, but it wasn't. My whole life, I had envisioned going to Washington to fight for something I believed in. This was the place you could change things. This was the place that made us unlike anywhere in the world. That's what I really believed. That's what I needed to believe.

But all around me, I was surrounded by pain. Parent after parent, red-faced from sweating and red-eyed from crying, was listening to the speeches somberly. Gathered together in that space, they put the magnitude of the disaster into focus. These weren't statistics. These children weren't collateral damage. They weren't faceless families we could feel sorry for and forget.

They were real. Real children, real parents, and real families devastated by what had happened to their children and their lives. And they were in terrible agony, angry about why and how it all happened, outraged at being dismissed, and desperate for help. And in response, they were being ridiculed and accused of hurting other children. It hurt in a way I can't fully describe.

To keep focused, I frequently scanned the crowd for familiar faces. So many of the people I had come to know online had made the journey to DC to speak out on their child's behalf. When Jenny asked us to hold our pictures of our affected children in the air and turn around to face the media, I thought I would lose it. I stared at the ground beneath me instead.

Eventually, the rally came to a close, and a long line formed under a tree to take a picture with Jenny and Jim. I helped corral those who wanted a photo and caught up with some of my friends I hadn't been able to speak with yet. It was then I saw my friend Michelle.

Michelle and I had met online years before. She was one of the first mothers I remembered meeting in the chat rooms, and she was a sweetheart. The first time I went to DC for a rally, she and I and another friend shared a room together.

I liked Michelle a lot. She was beautiful and had the prettiest Southern accent. She also had a daughter who was affected. We—mothers of daughters on the spectrum—are far outnumbered, so finding her was a blessing.

Today, however, I was nervous to see her. I was also surprised. I didn't think she would be able to make it or handle it. Her daughter had wandered away from her at a family party the month before. She made it to the neighbor's pool and drowned before anyone found her.

I approached her cautiously and tried to avoid looking at the picture of her beautiful little girl in the photo. I couldn't. It seared into my brain while we tearfully embraced, and all of the panic and anxiety I felt when Emma wandered out of our hotel room came back. I easily could have been Michelle. Why I wasn't, I'll never know.

The rally received some coverage, but it didn't make that much of a difference. Some members of the media even used it as a way to make fun of us. One journalist, an author, staunch defender of vaccines, and staunch critic of parents like me, came arguably for the purpose of harassing us.

I remember him smiling on the side of the Mall as we gathered that morning, trying to get people to engage with him. Most didn't. We knew full well he thought we were a joke.

"Ah yes, this is so funny," I remember thinking as I stared at him. "Hilarious. Dead kids, government lies, and brain injury are so hysterical."

But I also remember someone else on the Mall that morning: a cute guy about my age wrapped in camera gear, wearing the same shirt as me, carrying a huge microphone with a furry thing over it.

He was making a movie, someone told me. His name was Eric, and he had been poisoned by Thimerosal, too, only he was twenty-nine years old when it happened.

I was intrigued and anxious to talk to him. For the first time, an adult could tell us how it felt. And for the first time, our story would be put on film. I tried to find him to no avail. I wouldn't actually meet him or see his film for another six years.

Chapter 11

Opposition—Organized Medicine Strikes Back

For over seventy years, the medical community has blamed mothers for autism. From the very first diagnoses given at John Hopkins University in the early 1940s, Dr. Leo Kanner, the first doctor to name to the disorder, looked to parents as the cause.

Dr. Kanner was the world's leading authority on childhood psychiatry at the time. In 1935, he wrote a textbook called *Child Psychiatry* in which he identified and described every childhood psychiatric disorder known at the time. At the time of its publication, he was working at Johns Hopkins University Hospital in Baltimore, Maryland, where he had been since 1928. It was here the first children in the world to present with autism would come, and he was the reason they did.

At the time of the book's publication, Dr. Kanner was forty-nine years old, had lived on two continents, and had worked at another psychiatric hospital prior to writing the following words in a paper published in the medical journal *The Nervous Child* in April 1943. His words remain at the center of the debate to this day: "Since 1938, there have come to our attention a number of children whose condition differs so markedly and uniquely from anything reported so far, that each case merits—and, I hope, will eventually receive—a detailed consideration of its fascinating peculiarities."

His statement was extraordinary. As a leading authority on child psychiatry who had just written an exhaustive, authoritative textbook for all known psychiatric conditions affecting children only eight years earlier, he was clearly stating that autism was *new*. Furthermore, he claimed, it was *peculiar* and began to show up around 1938.

If Dr. Kanner was right, autism cannot be a genetic disorder. Something in the environment had to be causing it, something new in the 1930s that children across the country were being exposed to for the first time.

Unfortunately, however, as a psychiatrist in the age of Sigmund Freud, even though he actually rejected much of Freudian theory, he did not look to the literal environment as the cause. He looked instead to the emotional environment, the one in which a child would be nurtured.

He looked to the parents, and he looked to see how they could be responsible. Due to their high levels of education, intelligence, and their careers (mostly scientists, doctors, teachers, and researchers), he theorized, they were cold and clinical. In his mind, it was likely they were subconsciously more attached to their careers than their children. He even coined the phrase "refrigerator parents" to describe them.

The children had no choice but to turn inward, giving themselves the love and care their parents did not, the rationale went. They created a world of their own to cope in, Kanner believed—the word *autism* comes from the Greek word for "self," *autos*, suggesting complete self-absorption.

This is how and why autism became known as a psychiatric condition, as well as how and why it remains in that category today. Even though he also believed that children were born autistic, which made his theories about parental responsibility confusing at best,

Dr. Kanner said that's what happened. Because he was the world's leading authority, everyone believed him.

Over time, the theory grew even worse. At first, both mothers and fathers were blamed for this detachment disorder, but eventually it became only the mother's fault. By 1967, unbelievably, it was no longer just that these mothers didn't love their children; another autism researcher named Bruno Bettelheim out of the University of Chicago suggested they were actually homicidal.

Not only did they resent their children, he believed, they actually wanted to kill them. That summer, he published a book called *The Empty Fortress* all about his theory, to great praise. The *New York Times* even picked it as a top summer read. And in 1981, he was quoted as saying, "All my life, I have been working with children whose lives were destroyed because their mothers hated them."

But by the 1980s, another autism researcher and father of an affected child, Dr. Bernard Rimland, quashed that theory once and for all. He knew his wife was anything but cold and aloof, let alone homicidal, and he dedicated his career to putting that theory to bed. He was profoundly successful in doing so, too. Dr. Rimland's contribution to our understanding and treatment of autism is nothing short of heroic.

Even so, the medical community's decades of misogynistic theories of causation caused profound damage. I have no doubt the neurologist we visited in 2004 had been taught Kanner and Bettelheim's theories. He in all likelihood accused me of being disappointed in Emma, thereby causing or exacerbating her problems, because he was very likely taught that that was what happened.

And although it's wonderful that those views have been appropriately relegated to the garbage bin, we haven't quite taken out the trash yet. Now, instead of mothers being blamed for their emotional flaws, they are being blamed for their genetic ones instead. Likewise, they are being blamed for circumstantial environmental causes.

Too much television. Not talking to their children. Being depressed. Being old. Being fat. Marrying geeks. Marrying depressed geeks. Marrying old depressed geeks. These are only some of the proposed causes recently researched, published, and suggested as the real culprits behind the autism epidemic.

So truly, not much has changed in the almost eighty years since Kanner's first wrong turn. Moms are still the problem. Moms are still the cause. And moms are still to blame.

"You caused a mental condition in your child," the medical community has claimed about mothers for over seven decades.

"No, *you* caused a *medical* one," mothers have finally fired back at them.

For the first time since the discovery of autism, mothers have turned the tables. They weren't the ones to cause their child's autism, they realized, especially as the numbers of them sharing their stories exploded, *doctors* were. And for the first time, doctors were going to see what it felt like to be on the receiving end of such a strong accusation.

It's fair to say, they don't like it either.

The doctors

The perfect example of this hostility can be witnessed by watching a few minutes of an episode of *The Doctors* that aired in May 2009. Jenny McCarthy appeared with her son's doctor, Dr. Jerry Kartzinel, to discuss autism. Dr. Kartzinel is also the father of an affected child and now dedicates his practice to helping children on the spectrum.

Jenny and Dr. Jerry shared the stage with the other regular doctors of the show, Dr. Jim Sears and Dr. Travis Stork. In the audience was Generation Rescue's founder, J.B. Handley. When the discussion got heated and J.B. scolded Dr. Stork to "read the science" being used to confirm vaccine safety, Dr. Stork lost his cool.

"All you're doing is antagonizing a medical community that wants to help these children!" he shouted.

He was flustered, angry, and highly defensive. That anyone would accuse him or his colleagues of harming children in the name of trying to help was offensive and outrageous.

"Good," I smirked as I watched him come undone. "Now you know how it feels."

Autism's false Offit

Dr. Paul Offit was happy to take up the cause and champion the defense of doctors, immunizations, and medicine as the accusations against them took hold. He was having none of it. Doctors were the innocent victims of autism, he implied, the real folks who had children's best interests at heart.

He has recently gone so far as to suggest that if you won't love your child enough to vaccinate him, he and his colleagues will. He is also instrumental in the aggressive attempt to eliminate personal and religious belief exemptions to vaccines throughout the country. And he has encouraged all pediatricians to fire noncompliant vaccine parents from their practices, several of whom are now doing so.

Shame. Threats. Name-calling. Belittling. Coercion. Banishment. These are all a big part of the defensive playbook.

Moreover, Dr. Offit positioned himself as the authority on all things autism in a series of books on the topic. He received tremendous praise for them and was later given an award by the American Academy of Pediatrics for putting himself in the proverbial line of fire.

According to Dr. Offit, doctors didn't do anything wrong. Irresponsible parents using snake oil and scaring people away from vaccines were the true villains of the autism epidemic. He was quite successful in flipping the paradigm to suggest we were not only wrong but also legitimately dangerous.

He has since become the main voice against the "anti-vaccine" movement. He is also frequently on television, in the newspapers, and in the media as the authority on autism, vaccines, and the controversy. With little acknowledgement of his shortcomings and conflicts, he has had the stage for some time.

What most people don't know, however, is that Dr. Offit has never treated a single child with autism. Many doctors speak out against the correlation between vaccines and autism, but have no expertise with autism. As always, they have no idea what causes the disorder, they just know it isn't them.

Dr. Offit is also a vaccine patent holder. He holds the patent on an anti-diarrhea vaccine that was purchased by Merck. Estimates are that he made millions from it.

Nonetheless, Dr. Offit continues to be a vaccine industry spokesperson. And along with a host of other doctors, authors, journalists, and even celebrities (because as long as you say vaccines are great, being a celebrity doesn't matter), he maintains the positions

- that there is no evidence to link vaccines to autism;
- that Jenny McCarthy and Andrew Wakefield are responsible for the fact anyone thinks there is;
- that the science to disprove such a link is reliable, exhaustive, and solid;
- that vaccine injury is extraordinarily rare and when it happens, it is acceptable;
- that personal liberty does not trump public health;
- that failing to vaccinate a child is child abuse and criminal neglect;
- that doctors know better than parents;
- that autism has been around forever;
- that mercury has absolutely nothing to do with it;
- that medically treating autism is dangerous; and
- that doctors have just gotten better at diagnosing autism, which is why we think there's an epidemic, but there's not.

That's their story, and they are sticking to it.

The original 11

But facts are funny things, especially historical ones. Scientific "facts" can be generated. Studies can be designed to conclude with desired outcomes. Science can be manipulated, data stratified, and evidence thrown away when it doesn't fit the narrative of the people paying for it. Americans know this, and I would argue, have even come to expect it.

This is the reason so many people no longer trust "science" as the all-knowing, all-powerful authority it once was. Science and scientists—most people have lived through several examples in their lives by now—can easily be corrupted. Tobacco, Vioxx, and all of the legal commercials that happen to pop up a few years after a new miracle drug hits the market prove it.

In these cases, historical evidence, which cannot be changed, only interpreted, becomes perhaps even more important than scientific evidence. When historical fact contradicts scientific fact regarding the exact same instance, one of them has to be wrong. It is the equivalent of having conclusive video evidence of a criminal in the act, but a DNA test concluding it isn't the criminal in the video. The DNA test has to be wrong, especially if it turns out the criminal's best friend ran the test. In my opinion, this conflict is profound when it comes to autism.

In addition to identifying autism as a new problem and giving it a name, the world's leading authority on childhood psychiatry, Dr. Kanner, kept detailed records on the first eleven cases that presented to him. Like other psychiatrists of the day, he used a first name and last initial to refer to his patients in order keep them anonymous.

Dan Olmsted and Mark Blaxill decided to find these first eleven children, and with the help of Teresa Conrick, a friend and the mother of an affected child, were successful in uncovering the identities of eight of them. The story of how they did it, along with the history and evidence of what I've described regarding Kanner and autism, is detailed in their book, *The Age of Autism: Mercury, Medicine, and a Man-made Epidemic.*

They hypothesized Kanner had made one very big wrong turn when he theorized about the causation of autism. He wasn't wrong that it was new, and he wasn't necessarily wrong about the significance of the parents' occupations, intelligence, or education, they argued. It was something that stood out as important.

What he was wrong about, they suggested, was the significance of this information. Perhaps autism wasn't caused by the emotional coldness of high-achieving professionals who worked; perhaps it was what they worked *with*.

As mentioned earlier, the man-made ethyl mercury compound created by chemical engineer Morris Kharasch in the 1920s was patented and commercialized before the existence of the FDA to check for safety. Three of the new products included a seed preservative, a lumber preservative, and a biologics preservative.

DuPont filed a trademark application on May 13, 1929, for an ethyl mercury fungicide called Ceresan, teaming up with German corporation Bayer (who was also in the fungicide business), to market it here and abroad.

DuPont also purchased the rights to the lumber preservative and released Lignasan in 1930. And Eli Lilly purchased the rights to the biologics preservative named Merthiolate (now called Thimerosal) in 1928.

By the end of 1931, all three products were in commercial use in very specific locations. Thimerosal was placed in the new diphtheria toxoid vaccine and was first used in Baltimore, Maryland, that year.

Plant pathologists experimented with Ceresan, including at universities. By the end of the 1930s, it had been used on tobacco, cotton, tomatoes, and cabbage. And Lignasan, the lumber preservative, had been put to the test in three specific lumberyards before its widespread use, two in Mississippi and one in Louisiana.

Case No.	Name	Birthdate	From	Father	Mother
Child 1	Donald T.	9/8/33	Forest, Mississippi	Lawyer	Teacher
Child 2	Frederick W.	5/23/36	Madison, Wisconsin	Plant Pathologist	Teacher
Child 3	Richard M.	11/17/37	North Carolina	Forestry Professor	Teacher
Child 4	Paul G.	1935		Engineer	
Child 5	Barbara K.	10/30/33	Baltimore, Maryland	Psychiatrist	Nurse
Child 6	Virginia S.	9/13/31	Baltimore, Maryland	Psychiatrist	
Child 7	Herbert B.	11/18/37	Baltimore, Maryland	Psychiatrist	Pediatrician
Child 8	Alfred L.	6/20/32	Baltimore, Maryland	Patent Examiner	Psychologist
Child 9	Charles N.	8/9/38		Clothing Merchant	Theater Agent
Child 10	John F.	9/19/37	Baltimore, Maryland	Psychiatrist	Pathology Lab Stenographer
Child 11	Elaine C.	2/3/32		Copywriter	Editor

These are the names, birthdates, origins, and parental occupations of the first eleven children to visit Dr. Kanner from 1938 to 1943 and eventually be diagnosed with autism, and the order in which he presented them.

Psychiatry as a profession of so many of the fathers of these children seems significant. While it may be argued they would be the folks most likely to recognize a problem in their children and seek help where they worked, there is something else to consider.

Psychiatry at that point in time often used mercury to treat a form of insanity. Prior to antibiotic use, "general paralysis of the insane," commonly known as GPI, was an affliction approximately 10 to 15 percent of syphilis sufferers developed later in life. GPI was often deadly, but prior to death, struck its victims with delusions of grandeur, episodes of mania, and more. It was, quite frankly, a horrific way to die.

Olmsted and Blaxill provide ample evidence to suggest that GPI was actually a "disease of the remedy." The mercury being used to treat the syphilis bacteria appeared to allow both access to the brain, causing a much worse problem.

That only white men seemed to be developing the condition was in fact the reason for the famous Tuskegee experiment. It didn't occur to doctors that perhaps the reason black men weren't getting GPI had nothing to do with their race, but rather because they couldn't afford the mercury used to treat the condition.

Additionally, as doctors working in Baltimore, Maryland, it is highly probable they were among the first to vaccinate their children with the new diphtheria toxoid vaccine released there, especially since Johns Hopkins University was an integral part of the effort to make it happen.

Olmsted and Blaxill were also the first to find child 1, Donald Triplett, in 2005. More importantly, they were the first to uncover the evidence that after being treated for his juvenile rheumatoid arthritis with gold salts, his autism symptoms improved. Authors

Caren Zucker and John Donvan hypothesize in their book *In a Different Key* that his remarkable success in life is due to his mother and the love and support of the community where he lived.

That his wooden house built in 1930 was very likely constructed with the lumber that was very likely treated with Lignasan, which had first been tested not far away from where his home was built, has been ignored.

Zucker and Donovan have also ignored his treatment with injectable gold salts for his rheumatoid arthritis as a possible reason for his improvement. The first person in the world ever diagnosed with autism, according to his own brother, *recovered from autism* when treated medically for arthritis. In his brother's words: ". . . the nervousness and extreme anxiety that had heretofore afflicted him all but disappeared. He became more social. . . . It was the most amazing thing I've ever seen. . . . He just had a miraculous response to the medicine."

Olmsted and Blaxill also discovered that two of the fathers of the first eleven children worked at the same university at one time. In 1963, William Miller and Frederick Wellman, complete and total strangers, linked only by the fact that they had two of the first three boys ever to be diagnosed with autism *in the world*, both happened to teach at North Carolina State University . . . and both happened to study ethyl mercury compounds as a part of their research—Miller in trees and Wellman in plants.

They also discovered Dr. Elizabeth Peabody Trevett, the mother of child 7. She was one of the original pioneers of the well-baby visit, an actual face and name behind the reason all parents go to the doctor when they do. The irony and tragedy of her legacy, if true, is jaw dropping.

She dedicated her life to vaccination, the reason for a well-baby visit to begin with, claiming a child "couldn't be vaccinated early enough or often enough" with diphtheria toxoid vaccine . . . that she happened to be responsible for administering . . . in Baltimore, Maryland . . . in the 1930s.

And then there was Vivian Murdock, the very first person born in the world ever to be diagnosed with autism, who was given up to an institution by her parents at the age of six. They, too, lived in Baltimore, Maryland. Vivian was born there . . . in 1931.

And perhaps the biggest smoking gun of all is the file of Frederick Wellman, father of child 4, a plant pathologist experimenting with mercury compounds on cabbage at the University of Wisconsin. Dan and Mark accessed his archives while doing research for their book. When they opened it, a brochure for Ceresan was right on top.

The media muddles the truth

Along with Dr. Offit's defensive response, coupled with the ignorance of these historical facts, other journalists and celebrities joined the fight to defend modern medicine. That autism was something to be cured, prevented, or treated became offensive. Then the idea that autism is even a problem became questioned. Today, the idea autism is an epidemic is being challenged.

Books like *The Panic Virus* by Seth Mnookin became best sellers. He argued that there was no merit to the theory vaccines had anything to do with autism and that everyone had simply panicked, nothing more than a powerful lesson in how not to overreact.

Later, there was Eula Bliss's book, *On Immunity*. In beautiful academic prose, she detailed how she came to believe that vaccines had nothing to do with anything causative regarding today's childhood epidemics of allergies, autoimmunity, and spectrum disorders. Mark Zuckerberg, of Facebook fame, promoted her book as an important read.

There was also journalist Brian Deer, who is attributed with exposing Dr. Wakefield as a fraud through a series of articles he wrote for Rupert Murdoch's *Times* of London. By the end of the decade, Wakefield had been "discredited." Deer received awards for his reporting.

Dr. Nancy Snyderman got visibly angry on the *Today Show* when confronted by Matt Lauer about parents questioning the role of vaccines in causing autism. Anderson Cooper and George Stephanopoulos looked like their heads were going to explode when they interviewed Andy Wakefield. A correspondent on CNN even scolded parents in 2015 to "Hear this well! Vaccines do not cause autism!"

Bloggers and Facebook pages appeared for the purpose of shaming vaccine-concerned parents. Celebrities also jumped in. Actress Amanda Pete called parents who don't vaccinate "parasites" (she later apologized). Other celebrities, like Penn and Teller, created skits to make fun of parents who suspected a vaccine–autism link, not so subtly titled "Bullshit!"

Years later with the measles scare, Jimmy Kimmel would do something similar on *Live!,* his late show. The same year, actress Kristen Bell would pen a *Huffington Post* article to proclaim that vaccines save lives and it is unacceptable not to vaccinate your kids.

Making fun of, bullying, ostracizing, and chastising parents with vaccine safety concerns and sick children became a sport over the last ten years. By 2015, the talking points were well versed and often spoken. Vaccines do not cause autism and only save lives; ergo, anyone who even implies they are dangerous, or that the science to defend them is untrustworthy, kills babies.

Frustrating to those of us on the inside was that many people in the mainstream were trivializing a very serious issue they really didn't seem to know a lot about.

Any honest person could see the science proclaiming a disproven link was suspicious. It used theoretical exposure rates, came up with questionable conclusions, and had tremendous conflicts of interest.

Any honest person could see that it only looked at one vaccine and one vaccine ingredient to exonerate the totality of the vaccine program, without considering vast exposures to mercury from outside sources, genetic vulnerability, mitochondrial dysfunction, or potential toxic synergy through pharmaceuticals, breast milk, pesticides, lead, aluminum, antibiotic, or acetaminophen exposure.

Any honest person could see that we were literally arguing over whether or not a synthetic form of organic mercury that had never been properly tested for safety caused the symptoms of mercury poisoning in children who were vulnerable to its effects.

Any honest person could see that the number of historical, biological, and anecdotal coincidences we were being asked to believe was extraordinary and, frankly, defied logic.

But that seemed to be the crux of the issue, I realized after a while . . . any *honest* person.

Chapter 12

Devastation—When Later Came

In July 2009, my college roommates and I arranged to spend a weekend together at my parents' lake house. The eight of us had been extremely close for years, but now that most of us were married and had children, it was harder to see one another. We couldn't wait to relive some of our best memories as roommates and friends.

Facebook had only recently become a phenomenon for people my age, and not everyone was on it just yet. Although we knew the basics about one another's lives, we didn't know the intimate details like we once had. We sat around the sunroom one afternoon catching up over wine.

At one point, someone made a comment about how amazing all of our lives had turned out. We were so blessed to be where we were, she claimed. Everything had worked out for us. We all graduated, secured great jobs, and were getting married and starting families. We were doctors, teachers, lawyers, and mothers. We had a lot to be thankful for.

"I mean, we've had some bumps in the road, like you with Emma," she nodded at me sincerely and sympathetically, "but really, our lives are pretty amazing." Everyone agreed and raised their glasses in cheers.

My body froze at the comment. For a few moments I felt suspended in time, watching these women I love laugh, and smile, and joke just as we had fifteen years earlier. In so many ways we were the same, and yet in so many ways we weren't, or at least I wasn't. I didn't know that person from fifteen years ago anymore.

My friend's comment echoed in my ears as I tried to process what it meant. Was she acknowledging that Emma's situation was serious, or was she dismissing it as not that big of a deal? "A bump in the road," in my mind, is an expression you use to describe a minor issue, a small problem, or a little detour.

Nothing about what I had dealt with for almost eight years felt anything like that. It was the exact opposite. My life skidded suddenly and unexpectedly off the road, fell into a ditch, and now, bloodied and bruised, I had to get my family, my car, and myself back up on it alone. I was exhausted, frightened, and traumatized.

A bump in the road? My God, no.

I excused myself to the bathroom where I contemplated how to move forward with the rest of the day. I was logical enough to know that my friend meant no harm. She's a wonderful and caring person whom I love dearly.

But I stared at my reflection as I relived all of the terror. The regression. The hotel escape. The ambulance ride. The weak episode. The neurologist. The blood draws. The doctors. The rallies. The bullies. My friend's dead child. I couldn't even talk about Emma without crying.

I shook my head side to side and took a deep breath. Breathing was something I had always been able to do to center myself. That and running were the only things that were keeping me sane.

But lately, they weren't doing the trick as they once had. No matter how much I was running, I wasn't able to feel at peace afterward.

And no matter how hard I was trying to center myself with my breath, it wasn't working either.

I had noticed about a year earlier that there seemed to be tightness in my chest, like a fist in the middle of it, that wouldn't dissipate no matter how hard I tried. I simply could not draw in a breath all the way. And one day, folding laundry, I found myself barely able to breathe, shaking ever so slightly, unable to calm down over nothing.

"Why am I so afraid all the time?" I shouted, aggravated, to no one in my bedroom. "What is wrong with me?"

I was angry with myself, insecure in a way I had never been before. Whatever it was, I couldn't place it.

So I started running more. Although I wasn't running competitively, I would easily run three- to five-mile routes several times a week. I always ran the same streets, and I always tried to finish strong. In high school track, we were trained to do so. You never gave up at the end of route; you gave it your all.

But that was becoming problematic, too. For the first time since running long distances in junior high, I was having a hard time "finishing strong." Every time I would sprint the last quarter mile around the bend to my home, I would burst into tears when I crossed my imaginary finish line. Not just a little crying, either. I'm talking a whole body sob, something so powerful that one time at the health club, it knocked me off the treadmill onto the floor.

People thought I had hurt myself physically, wondering if I had twisted an ankle. I let them think that. I was embarrassed to tell anyone that pushing myself to the brink physically was pushing me to the brink emotionally. I thought I was going crazy.

Phobias that had started around then didn't help. In 2007, as a ten-year anniversary present, I took Mike to see Croatia play England at Wembley Stadium in London for the European Cup qualifying game. On the way out of the stadium, amidst tens of thousands of people walking down one gigantic, yet enclosed, walkway, I became terrified.

For the first time ever, I was afraid of a crowd. I made my way over to the wall where I could see a way out and looked at the ground to stay focused. On the "Tube," the subway system in London we took back to our hotel, I had to hold Mike's hand and count to one hundred over and over again to take my mind off of the enclosed space jam-packed with people all around me.

I was not only terrified of the confined space, I was terrified of what was happening to me. I had been afraid of heights my whole life. Small spaces? Not really. And crowds? Not ever. For years, my friends and I watched fireworks in Grant Park, Chicago, with over a million other people.

The only thing that remained that I could do to cope with these powerful feelings was to write. Writing had always been my most important outlet. When I wrote, I was free. When the words got put on paper, it was as if I was expelling them out of my body.

So I came home after the girls' weekend and crafted a blog post about the experience. "A Bump in the Road," it was called, and it became one of the most popular posts I have ever written. In detail and with brutal honestly, I shared how I felt, what the conversation in my head went like in the bathroom, and how I had come to believe that most people truly couldn't understand what it was like to experience regressive autism.

It was the equivalent of losing a child that was still alive, I believed, an expression I heard a father of an affected child once use. The baby girl I brought into the world was now not able to experience life in the way that God intended. A stupid, unnecessary, terrible mistake, I was convinced, took her health, her intelligence, and her ability to function socially in the world as she should have.

Was she alive? *Yes.* Was I grateful for that? *Of course.* Was she as severe and low functioning as she could have been? *Not even close.* We had so much to be thankful for.

But we had so much to be heartbroken over, too. By 2009, in third grade, Emma was falling further and further behind academically and socially. She went from having no aide in kindergarten or first grade, to being placed in a small self-contained reading and math class for most of the day. Although necessary, it isolated her from her typical peers, with whom she still had a hard time connecting without assistance.

More worrisome, her social immaturity was getting her bullied. She still picked her nose whenever she felt like it, regardless of when or where she was. She got teased all the time. And because she couldn't keep up conversationally with the other kids about their interests and such, as she was still developmentally several years younger and still mildly speech delayed, she would compensate by acting silly and strange. Kids laughed at her, not with her.

Every day my heart broke for all of these reasons and more. I had so naively thought that a few years of hard work at the beginning of our journey would equate to being able to put autism behind us. In 2009, I had worked tirelessly for almost five years. I wanted it to be over. I was so done with the extreme highs and lows. One minute grateful simply for the fact she could speak, the next minute furious she couldn't do it well. It felt like being thrashed about on a raft in the ocean.

Not only that, there was there no way to get justice, I finally realized around that time. I was lucky if I could even get people to believe me!

People knew how to gauge the seriousness of cancer. They didn't know how to gauge autism. By then, the movement to normalize it, accept it, and embrace it as a difference, not a disability, had begun. I even received hate mail telling me I should be ashamed of myself for being so upset about Emma's autism.

The message was becoming clearer by the day. I shouldn't tell people what happened to us. I shouldn't talk about my concerns about why it happened. I shouldn't try to do anything about it. And now, I shouldn't even feel anything about it. I wasn't even entitled to experience or express my own pain without judgment.

Worst of all, there was no closure. There never would be, either. There would never be a day for as long as I lived that I didn't wonder, *what if?*

The feeling was unfathomable, wreaking havoc on my body, my marriage, and my life. To what extent, and how badly, I just didn't realize yet.

Blueberries and a bathroom

The following summer, Mike, the kids, and I took a vacation to Saugatuck, Michigan. Several friends and family members raved about the place, encouraging it as a family getaway. One of Mike's friends had a farm where we could stay. We decided to take the trip.

As everyone claimed, the town was beautiful. It sat east of Lake Michigan, providing a view I had never seen. For the first time, I watched the sun go down over it in the evening (something you cannot do in downtown Chicago).

We shopped, swam, ate in quaint cafes, and even took a wild trip on some dune buggies. By all accounts, it was a successful family vacation. The kids had fun, everyone got along, and it was relatively inexpensive. Emma was long past being nonverbal or in danger of eloping. Life was nothing like it had been. The last day, we even stopped to pick fresh blueberries and raspberries.

The photo album I put together of the trip, along with the family photo I used for that year's Christmas card, captured the images of a healthy, happy family having a wonderful time. It's sunny, we're all smiling, and everyone appears to be having fun. What it doesn't show, however, is my truth.

Every day of that trip I struggled to get out of bed. If there were a dial on my chest, one that could be turned to the right to give you more energy, and one that could be turned to the left to take it all away, mine was as far left as it could go. All joy, motivation, and concern for anyone or anything disappeared. Every ounce of what I had left in me was just enough to go through the motions of my life.

I sat in the passenger side of the minivan as Mike drove, lifeless, mostly speechless, and distant. A few times, I caught myself thinking, I could just open this door right now and roll out as we speed along the highway.

I was careful not entertain those thoughts for long, or so I believed. I'd had weird thoughts like that once before. After my son was born, my sleep deprivation in combination with post-partum depression started to mess with my mind. Later, when Brooke Shields went public with her struggle, I took comfort in knowing I wasn't alone.

And so thinking a crazy thought like tossing myself out of a moving vehicle didn't seem as frightening as it once had. I knew not to take myself seriously. I knew it just meant I was depressed. Still, the recognition I was depressed didn't make it any easier not to feel it.

One night, as it rained heavily and loudly on our small cabin, I couldn't sleep. Anxiety crushed me as I desperately tried to count, breathe, and pray to relax. No matter how hard I tried, the incessant, guilt-ridden thoughts wouldn't go away.

"You did this to her," they taunted me.

"You. You stupid, stupid woman. You let it happen. You're the one that ignored your instinct. You're the one that wouldn't confront them when you suspected what was wrong. Imagine if you had!

"But you didn't, you scared piece of shit. You're going to hell, Julie. And you deserve it. You made life on earth hell for her. You better believe you're getting an afterlife in hell for it."

It felt like a dream, but it wasn't. The thoughts wouldn't go away no matter how much I tossed and turned. I finally lay face up staring at the ceiling fan in the lightning-lit room and let myself cry. The thunder masked my sobs along with the pillow I placed over my head.

When I stopped, I needed a tissue. My head hurt, my nose was running, and I was a mess. I carefully stepped through the small space filled with suitcases, shoes, and a blow-up mattress to make my way to the bathroom. Taking care not to wake anyone, I entered and closed the door behind me before turning on the light.

In the bathroom, I sat on the toilet with the lid down and put my head in my hands. To my right was a pink bathtub and sink with our shampoos, toothbrushes, toothpastes, and razors. It was then I got an idea.

I could kill myself, I realized looking at the razor blade. I should kill myself. Whoever was telling me I was responsible for Emma's suffering was right. It was my fault, and I deserved to die. It wasn't about stopping my pain, no. It was about getting what I deserved.

The part of me that knew this wasn't real, that I shouldn't even consider such a stupid idea, and that this was depression talking, not me, was there, but faint. Never in my life have I felt so desperate. Never in my life have I felt more guilty, more sorry, and more unworthy of living. It was powerful, a force at odds with all intellect I had . . . and it was winning.

I was just about to stand up when the bad thoughts started again.

"Oh, no," they said to me clearly. "You're not going out like that. The only way this will ever be equal is if your thoughts, your speech, your memories, your intellect, and your bodily functions all diminish like hers, and all while you stay conscious in the background of it happening. Unable to communicate your needs, you will die in silence without anyone knowing how you feel. That's how you're going to die, Julie. Only then will Emma have justice."

This was ridiculous, my sanity suddenly decided. I shook my head once again to fling the thought away, stood up, and splashed my face with water before heading back to bed.

"Alzheimer's," I realized, half smirking, half serious, just about to flick off the light switch.

"Son of a bitch, I'm going to die from Alzheimer's."

When later came

Part of the reason for my depression that year was the publication of Dan and Mark's book. At a conference that spring, I had received an early copy. Every year, they would take all of the contributing editors out to dinner as a thank-you for our contributions.

Within a few days, I devoured the almost 400-page book. Its evidence was extraordinary, in my view, worthy of the Nobel Prize. I immediately reached out to tell them so.

For if they were right, they had also discovered that we were living in a new era of disease. It was no longer appropriate to look to one germ, one virus, or one microbe as the cause. The real model for industrial disease, they argued, was one metal and one microbe. The combination, able to access the blood–brain barrier in a way impossible before the Age of Better Living through Chemistry, was responsible for today's plagues.

I still believe they are right, and I still believe that someday, hopefully in our lifetime, they will receive the credit they deserve. Unfortunately, they haven't. The agricultural, chemical, and medical industrial complexes have been hesitant to embrace a theory that blames them for today's chronic diseases. Go figure.

But in early 2010, prior to the book's official release, its findings hit me hard. To start, I learned that the commonly used symbol of the medical profession, the staff with the two snakes wrapped around it called the caduceus, was actually the symbol for the Roman god Mercury. (This is a common mistake in medicine. It should be the rod of Asclepius, with only one snake.) The irony crushed me. So did revisiting all of the possible sources and symptoms of exposure I had learned about years prior.

There were literally dozens of ways human beings could be affected by mercury. There were also dozens of ways you could be exposed to it. Our coal-burning plants, our dental fillings, our medicines, our over-the-counter products including skin-bleaching creams and eye drops, and, yes, our vaccines contained it. I knew all that.

But our fish did, too, something I had completely forgotten about until reading their book. Big fish like shark and swordfish were the worst offenders. As the mercury deposited in the oceans from coal burning, the bigger fish became the most toxic. In 2001 and 2004 the FDA had issued new safety guidelines about eating big fish because of the problem.

"Good thing I never eat that," I thought to myself reading all about it. And suddenly, just like that, I remembered.

Tuna. The work-out program. The wedding. Looking in the books. It all came flooding back. Why and how it had all been put out of my mind for that long, I'll never know. Denial, I suppose.

I leapt from the desk where I was reading and tore into the basement. On one wall, I had placed a bookshelf with all of my important parenting books, some of my fictional favorites, and several others I wanted at easy access. My psychology book from the University of Illinois was one of them. Around 1991, it claimed, autism was extremely rare, affecting at most 1 in 10,000 children worldwide.

My baby bibles, as I had referred to them, were there as well. I passed them over and frantically scanned the shelf beneath them. I needed to find the exercise book I had used in the summer of 2001. Maybe I was mistaken, I hoped. Maybe I really didn't eat it after all.

I found it and flipped anxiously to the section on the diet. Like I remembered, it offered only a few choices for protein, mostly eggs, chicken, or fish. I flipped to the back where it allowed you to write down what you had eaten each day. I knew I had been diligent about keeping track, just like I had for Emma's diet years later, but when I turned to those pages, they were empty.

I stood stupefied for a moment when I remembered I kept a separate journal. I ran over to the other part of the basement where I kept it. On the shelves there were also boxes of memories I had kept by year. I scanned them for 2001 when I found our family memory box and then one for Emma exclusively.

I brought them both over and set them on the floor, then went back to the other shelves with the binders. My heart raced as I searched frantically for the damaging evidence of my guilt. Now everything was making sense.

I knew I had a root canal while pregnant, but even that seemed unlikely to be the main cause. And only one series of her vaccines had Thimerosal. It was not near the amount other children had been exposed to, which didn't necessarily mean it wasn't implicated, but always struck me as important. This made sense. The tuna I ate. The tuna I had forgotten about. That had to be it.

I found the binder and held it for a second before opening it. In the moments it would take me to flip through the pages and confirm what I had done, my life would again change forever. Now it would be for certain. I had literally helped poison my child. Not just my doctors. Not just the government. Not just someone on the outside. Me.

I looked at the pages in fear, day after day, June 16, 2001 . . . June 17, 2001 . . . June 18, 2001 . . . all detailing the amount I had eaten. Some days one can, most days none. I checked and double checked. Contrary to what I had thought, it wasn't nearly as much as I had worried. And then I remembered that's because I fucking hate tuna. Of course I didn't eat that much.

If my notes were correct, I ate no more than a few cans a week in just over six weeks, far less than *What to Expect When You're Expecting* said was safe when you were pregnant. And, I remembered, I was only breastfeeding about half of the time at that point because of my breast infection.

According to the experts, it was highly unlikely she got a significant amount of mercury from that. But then I realized, maybe the amount they claimed was safe for the general population wasn't important. Maybe it was just enough to finally push *her* over the edge. Maybe it was just enough to combine with the antibiotics, aluminum, and acetaminophen in her system to get trapped and wreak havoc on her body.

That's the thing about mercury. It's sneaky. It's synergistic. And it affects everyone differently. It's a fallacy that a uniform "safe" amount exists for everyone. We simply do not know what that number is for every individual.

Whatever the truth was, it didn't matter in that moment. It was just another thing in a long line of unfortunate coincidences that went wrong for us where medicine, mankind, and mercury were concerned.

That her autism was likely the result of listening to the experts, believing my regulators, trusting them to have my back and my daughter's, and following my doctor's advice, engulfed me in pain. I could no longer contain my rage. I took the binder and flung it across the basement.

"AGHHH!!!!!" I screamed in agony. A swell of emotion, a combination of fury and heartbreak, filled my body and took over my mind. I lost control.

"AGHHHH!!!!" I screamed again as I ran back to the shelves with my baby bibles.

"You!" I held up the "authoritative" book on development from the American Academy of Pediatrics. "You don't even have the words *mercury* or *autism* in here, you piece of shit book!" I threw it on the ground.

"And you!" I held up *What to Expect When You're Expecting*. "You tell me eating tuna fish from a can a couple of times a week should be fine! Should! Be! Fine!" I opened to the page and read it out loud sarcastically.

"Well, it's not fine!" I tossed it across the room. "It's! Not! Fine!"

I raced to the box of memories on the floor and opened them carelessly. On the top of Emma's box was her baby book, only partially filled out, except the back pages where I documented her illnesses. When your child stops developing normally, the last thing you want to do is document it. Most of the pages were empty. The book was far more painful than pleasant.

The folder we got from the hospital with her first photos lay under it. I opened it to see the image of her beautiful, angelic face, perfectly colored, perfectly healthy, captured with her eyes closed. The woman who had tried to get her to wake just couldn't. It was adorable.

The proofs had come with a variety of backgrounds you could choose from when you ordered. There were balloons, hearts, and puzzle pieces as options. Yes, staring right back at me was a picture of my newborn daughter surrounded by puzzle pieces, the well-known symbol of autism, with "PROOF" stamped across her face.

"Oh, this is *funny*, God!" I cackled loudly as I held the pictures in the air. I was kneeling, surrounded by books, papers, memories, and the broken dreams I had left in my destructive path.

"Really fucking funny, *God*!" I began to laugh, but not a good laugh, a crazy laugh—the kind of laugh a crazy person makes that frightens you. Within a few seconds, it morphed to a sob. Shortly thereafter, it was a wail. With my hair matted to my face, a sound came out of me I didn't know I could make. It felt like I was being cracked in half.

Unable to stand, or breathe, I surrendered to the pain that enveloped me whole on the basement floor. There was no getting out of it. There was no putting it off, no fighting through it, no scheduling it for another day, another time, another moment. It was here, under the surface the whole time, waiting to come spilling out, showing itself in bad dreams, anxiety, depression, and phobias.

Grief. Real, pure, utter grief took me over in that space and time. I had never felt anything like it, and I have never felt anything like it since. Later, I remembered saying the time when I would eventually let myself cry about it had finally come.

The state of our union

The housing crisis hit us hard, as it did millions of other Americans. The house we built in 2005 was worth significantly less than what we paid for it by 2012. Our neighborhood, which we had picked based on the promise that a joint park was being put in with another development, had simply stopped in time.

There was no park and no development. The school that was supposed to be built within walking distance was never built, either. The two lots remain empty to this day.

The housing collapse had other far-reaching effects that seeped into my career. For years after Emma's diagnosis, I requested to work part time. Even teaching one less class than a full load freed up enough time to get her back and forth to therapies and work with her academically. An incorrectly formatted seniority list misled me for years into thinking I had the job security to choose that. Even after bringing it to the attention of my administrators and union, I was assured I was safe to do so.

Alas, I was not. And by 2011, with a change in administration, the mistake was brought to everyone's attention. I was outraged and encouraged to sue, but I didn't have it in me to take on another fight. By 2012, I lost my teaching position at the high school where I had worked for fourteen years. They, too, were in a financial crisis.

At home, Mike and I were at odds. The stress of our financial situation, my job situation, and the years of dealing with autism were pulling us apart. Whereas I went out with my pain, he went in. Whereas I found a new group of friends to fight this battle and heal my child, he isolated himself from everyone instead, including me.

It happened slowly, but by fall of 2012, our marriage was seriously hurting. In many ways, we lived separate lives. I had close relationships with people he had never met. I traveled to conferences alone and spoke or wrote publicly about our lives, usually without asking. For years, I wanted to believe that because he never said it bothered him, it didn't. I had no idea whether I was right or to what extent.

Likewise, I had no idea how much pain he was in. Mike never showed much emotion regarding Emma's autism. He was always "fun daddy," the light of her life, wrestling with her on the floor and taking her to the park, the store, and wherever he could to enjoy their time together. When I asked him about it, he wouldn't say much.

"It is what it is" is about the extent to which he would explain. It seemed so easy for him. There was nothing he could do about the past, he said. It happened, and now we needed to move forward and take care of it. For him, it was that simple.

Or so I thought. I didn't realize the pressure he was putting on himself to care for his little girl. I didn't know that he spent his nights awake wondering who would take care of her after we were gone. I didn't know he was terrified that men would take advantage of her as she got older. That thought hadn't ever occurred to me.

So I didn't know that he was taking aggressive chances with our retirement account in an effort to make some big gains. I didn't know until the day he did it that he purchased a foreclosure to flip. And I didn't know he was slipping into a depression, right in front of my face; I was too occupied with my own pain to really notice or help.

All of his efforts failed. The retirement account was worth half of what it had been. The flip flopped. Worse, he borrowed money from his parents to do it. We owed them, too. We were now significantly worse off than we had been only five years earlier, and we would be for some time as we recovered. The stress began to choke us.

In 2012, we had to face another hard decision. Emma was now in sixth grade, and at that year's IEP, the special education director made a comment that changed everything for me.

"She'll have a good life," she dismissed me when I asked about Emma's future. Since third grade, her learning disabilities had become clear. College, which had been my ultimate goal, wasn't looking likely.

This was the director's reply when I asked if she thought Emma could ever go on to higher education. *No* would have been a better answer. This one felt patronizing. A "good life" wasn't good enough.

After the meeting, Mike and I had a tough discussion. In 2005, I started college savings plans for the kids. From my teaching salary, I put as much money as I could into them. If working meant they could go to college without debt, it was worth it.

I knew when we opened the plans that Emma was having problems. I knew that saving for her college tuition was perhaps not the best way to use our money right then. But I also knew I couldn't justify doing it for the other two and not her. It would be way too symbolic of what I believed her destiny would be if I didn't. I refused.

But now, her destiny seemed a little clearer. And the truth was it was a better use of our money if we closed her account. The program allowed a relative to purchase the plan if we wanted to sell it to them. If someone bought it, we would have enough to pay the other accounts in full. We knew it was the right thing to do.

It broke my heart. Although I understood the logic and the need, the thought of closing that account was devastating. I took a few months to finally decide to do it, and on January 24, 2012, I eventually sat down at our desk to fill out the paperwork.

Tears filled my eyes as I did, but I was careful not to let them show. The whole family was in the room with me watching the president's speech. He was making the State of the Union address that night.

I listened lightly, more intent on making sure I was signing things where they needed to be signed than listening to anything he had to say, when suddenly the president's words stopped me cold.

"I will not back down from protecting our children from mercury poisoning!" He stated forcefully, to much applause. I turned to the television in shock, not quite sure I had heard that right.

"What did he say?" I asked Mike to replay it. We listened again and looked at each other stunned.

"You have got to be kidding me," I laughed, disgusted, as I went back to selling Emma's college plan. "You have got to be fucking kidding me."

Light bulbs with mercury were a serious threat to children's safety, according to the president. Vaccines with mercury, however, were not. His administration even went so far as to call for the censorship of the conversation about it.

We sold Emma's plan that night. My brother purchased it, but not before reassuring me that he would always make sure she was taken care of. I know he means it, and I feel lucky to have him by my side.

But Mike took it differently. He had failed his little girl, he believed. Over and over again, he had failed to protect her, and now it seemed he was having a hard time providing for her.

He slipped further away from me that year, distant and sad, closed off and resentful. In November, after his fortieth birthday party, we got in an enormous fight.

Ten years to the day that Emma had the high-pitched screaming fit, arched her back, and stopped talking or smiling for months afterwards, I asked Mike to move out. We separated for the first time.

PART IV

THE RESULT

Chapter 13

Acceptance—Take a Walk

"A Bump in the Road" took on a life of its own. It was the first post I wrote that transcended the insulated autism community of which I was a part. My writing is and always has been for them. I accepted a long time ago that I wasn't always going to be believed, liked, or supported for my position. I was well aware of who my audience was.

So I didn't expect that post to do what it did. I was shocked as the "likes" and "shares" ticked up throughout the day, as well as over one hundred kind comments. I was even more shocked by the email I received. From around the world, parents, teachers, and therapists were thanking me for it. One commenter even called it "a masterpiece of grief and strength."

When I wrote it, I cried my eyes out. These days I can usually tell the emotional reaction I am going to get from people by using that as a measure, but at that time, I hadn't written enough to know that. I cried because it was my story and my pain. I did not expect it to provoke a reaction like that from anyone else.

I couldn't have been more wrong. Fellow autism moms still talk to me about it. One mom told me she printed it out and put it in her nightstand to read when she needs a good cry. And a psychologist asked me for my permission to use it as a part of her curriculum to explain the depth of despair and misunderstanding special-needs parents could feel.

I was flattered but very uncomfortable. That our story had seeped its way out of the protective bubble of our blog scared me. For a while, I decided it would be the last thing I would ever write about our life. I felt so vulnerable and exposed. I even felt obligated to apologize to my friends and family that I had included in it. In my honesty, I feared I hurt their feelings. "A Bump in the Road" might have been "A Toss Under the Bus" to them.

That anyone outside of the autism world would care what I had to say was surprising, to say the least. But they did care. A lot. And a friend of a childhood friend reached out to let me know. This person wanted to pay for private tutoring at a renowned reading school for Emma that summer based on what she had read.

She was not taking no for an answer, either, so I reluctantly but gratefully accepted. For weeks, we drove almost an hour both ways several days a week to give the expensive reading program a chance. Each drive, I learned a new lesson from the road.

I had to accept that although I had enemies, I had a lot of people in my corner. I wasn't nearly as alone as I thought. People weren't trying to hurt me with their ignorance about my pain either, I realized. They just really didn't know.

Which meant I might also need to accept that my biggest role in this issue would not be getting justice in the halls of Congress, changing laws or policy, or going on to become a politician, as my late grandmother predicted I would.

Perhaps the only thing I could really ever do to make a difference, I learned from writing that post, would be telling our story so that someone could do those things.

Rescue me

Within a year of the breakdowns in the basement and the bathroom, I noticed something. I could breathe. Just like that, out of the blue, I noticed I could take a deep breath. The knot in my chest, the tight fist that I felt for so long, was gone. I remember being so conscious of the change that I repeatedly kept taking deep breaths just to be sure.

Likewise, I was able to talk about Emma for the first time without crying or getting angry. For years, any mention of her progress, or lack thereof, any mention of the controversy, or God forbid, any mention of vaccines, would send me spiraling.

I had no patience to explain anything to anyone. I had no tolerance for people who read one paragraph of a biased article and thought they had an ounce of the knowledge I did. If my speech about any of those topics were visible, it would have been in ALL CAPS ALL THE TIME.

I was defensive, moody, angry, and anxious. I felt isolated, irritated, misunderstood, abandoned, and betrayed. But mostly, I was heartbroken.

Until one day, just like that, I wasn't. Gone was the persistent lump in my throat. Gone was the desire to rip someone's head off. Gone was the need to be right. I just cared a whole heck of a lot less than I ever had.

The freedom was astounding. Without the compulsion to convince the world of anything anymore, I was free to choose how to spend my time. I was free to choose the conversations I wanted to have. I was free to scroll past any post that denied or dismissed my life, my daughter, our experience, or our choices without getting in a long debate or discussion about it. I was free to write about other things in my life.

By breaking down, I had broken free. I was free. Free to choose to be more grateful than greedy. Free to accept my daughter for all that she was, not all that I had thought she was missing. Free to accept myself for having been through hell and survived. I was even free to run without crying.

In fact, I was free to walk if I wanted! For all the years since the marathon, I had been literally and figuratively running nonstop so far and so fast, determined never to slow down, never to stop, and always to finish strong.

Walking during a route, I had always felt, was the equivalent of being a quitter. I never walked. Ever. No matter how much I hurt or even if I had broken something, I always pushed through my pain . . . just like in Alaska.

It finally dawned on me, maybe it didn't matter if I ran everywhere or finished strong every day and every time. Maybe it just mattered that I moved at all. And maybe walking was not a sign of defeat, but a sign of strength.

Maybe slowing down and taking care of my pain, rather than running through it and from it all the time, only making it worse, was not only wiser, but also necessary. I have finally learned to take care of myself and walk whenever I need to.

I was also free to get back to doing what I loved. I loved to help other families affected by autism. I hadn't raised money in years to help others, so when another Chicago family starting doing so, I was thrilled.

Within a few years, they had taken a small gathering at a bar to a professionally thrown party with celebrities. They were raising hundreds of thousands of dollars. I was more than honored when they asked Mike and me to join them as co-hosts of the annual event. We eagerly accepted.

And so we joined the group of people responsible for putting on the annual Rescue Our Angels event in Chicago. The money raised goes toward a grant program offered by Generation Rescue. Families in financial need can apply to receive a grant that affords them the opportunity to work with a medical doctor specializing in helping children on the spectrum.

Without the doctors that helped us, I don't know where we would be. Raising money to help families gain the same medical care and raising awareness that for many, autism is treatable, preventable, and reversible, are the most important things I have ever felt I can do to help.

Other people had the same feelings. One of them happened to be a relative of rock-star legend and drummer of the Foo Fighters, Taylor Hawkins. A regular reader and mother of an affected child, she contacted *Age of Autism* with an offer. He was willing to do a concert for us, she claimed. His own band would put on a show to raise money in Los Angeles if we were interested.

Generation Rescue joined the efforts. Together, they arranged the evening at a club just off of Hollywood Boulevard. I vividly remember walking down the street in my jeans, high heels, and big hoop earrings anxious to experience a real rock and roll event in one of the places that defined the music of my generation.

Rolling Stone magazine was even there and did a nice write-up of the event afterward, which wasn't surprising. *Rolling Stone* has usually been good to us. Unlike *Salon,* they never retracted the article by Robert F. Kennedy, Jr., on the controversy.

Dan Olmsted and I spent most of our time with Taylor's family, enjoying the music and discussing our kids. And Taylor was gracious enough to spend time with all of us in between sets. It was an incredible night. He couldn't be a nicer guy.

For a long time, as I met celebrities and politicians through my activism, I felt guilty about it. Something about having these once-in-a-lifetime experiences because my daughter regressed into autism felt wrong. I often felt like I had to apologize or hide my experiences to avoid being judged.

But after I learned that it was only by fully accepting the depths of our pain that we could fully accept the blessings that came from them, I no longer worried about it. I thought I had learned that the day I met Oprah, but I hadn't. Yes, I got to meet a rock star. He even kissed me on the cheek.

And in the years to come, I would meet even more celebrities and work even more closely with some world-famous politicians and activists. It's been an incredible ride, for sure, but make no mistake: I would trade it all in a second, in a millisecond, for never having had a reason to meet any of them in the first place.

Last year, the Foo Fighters went on tour. As a part of it, they played to a sold-out Wrigley Field in Chicago. A fellow autism mom who has become a great friend over the years, and likewise, another mom of a little girl on the spectrum, had gotten tickets to the show.

That night, as it misted over the thousands of us dancing crowded together on the field, I looked around in awe at the meaning of that time and space for me. I was there because I had made a lifelong friend I would have never otherwise met had our children not had autism.

As the band broke into their famous song "Walk" and the crowd sang along loudly to the refrain, "I'm learning to walk again," I couldn't help but cry. This time, however, they were happy tears.

I had finally learned to walk again, that's for sure. I could even walk among the sea of people on that field without a worry in the world. My fear of crowds was finally gone.

Light it up true

By the end of the decade, Autism Speaks had become a force. It was and still is the leading organization for all things autism. With the millions of dollars it began with, coupled with the tens of millions more it was making from its walks, its Toys R Us campaign, and its celebrity comedy shows, Autism Speaks has been able to bring tremendous awareness to the world about autism.

Billboard campaigns, puzzle-piece logos, commercials, and media appearances to explain what autism was, what if anything could be done about it, and what new research was showing became common.

The month of April even became Autism Awareness month, and with it, buildings throughout the country lit themselves up blue to show support.

At first, the awareness campaign was a welcome one. Far too many families for far too long had to go through hell to get an answer about what was wrong with their child. Our story was a perfect example. The average age of diagnosis in the early 2000s was still four. By 2010, it was down to just before the age of three. Today, it is closer to two.

That was a great thing. Early intervention is key to helping a child recover and improve. The sooner you can start therapies of all kinds, the sooner you can make progress. It was wonderful to see such focus on the topic.

But by the early 2010s, the awareness message was morphing into something altogether new: acceptance. The panic and urgency with which autism had been treated the years prior was dwindling. Now, instead of being presented as an emergency and an epidemic, autism was being twisted into a difference, not a disability.

Likewise, the idea no parent should do anything to try and "change" or "cure" his or her child was born. Nonverbal, sensory-impaired, seizure-experiencing, tantrum-throwing, and socially inept, dependent children were gifts, this movement insisted. Suggesting otherwise was an insult. (Yes, our children are gifts, I agree, but no, their autism is not.)

Even the word "epidemic" became challenged. Some people have now taken the position there probably just isn't one. According to their view, autism is a natural state of the human condition, something that has been with us forever; we just didn't notice it, or call it that, or something.

They often point to the diagnostic change in the *Diagnostic and Statistical Manual of Psychiatric Disorders,* Fourth Edition, in 1994, to include Asperger's in the diagnosis as the cause for the increase in numbers. They almost always fail to mention, however, that according to the doctor who crafted the change, the changes were a "corrective narrowing" meant to make the autism diagnosis *harder* to get, not easier.

They also fail to mention that in the late fall of 1998, four years after the diagnostic change, the CDC canvassed every home and every child in Brick Township, New Jersey, for autism. A mother of recently diagnosed twins had done a survey of the schools and discovered that there were hardly any older children with the disorder.

When a group of parents organized to reach out to the CDC to tell them what they had found, they literally thought something might be in the water. So did the CDC, who went so far as to call it a "cluster."

To investigate, they unleashed a team of experts on the township and checked every single child age ten and under in it to count the autism numbers. They started in September and were ready to report by the end of January 1999. These are the rates of full syndrome autism they discovered:

Birth Year	Age	Rate (per 1,000)
1995	3 years old	2.5
1994	4 years old	6.1
1993	5 years old	7.8
1992	6 years old	7.0
1991	7 years old	6.4
1990	8 years old	2.0
1989	9 years old	0.0
1988	10 years old	0.0

It turned out there was not a single child nine or ten years old in Brick Township, New Jersey, born in 1988 or 1989, that had full syndrome autism, as determined by the CDC in the fall of 1998. Not a single one.

When they reported on the findings, however, the CDC did an interesting mathematical trick. By unevenly grouping the children in the ages of three to five years old and comparing them to children ages six to ten years old, they were able to report there was no statistically significant difference in the rate of autism between the groups.

It was a ridiculous comparison to make, using completely uneven groups, and the only possible way to twist the numbers to make such a case. Any honest examination of those numbers clearly shows there's a problem. And they were well aware that three-year-olds shouldn't be counted as an accurate reflection of their autism, as they likely didn't have a diagnosis yet.

In the words of Olmsted and Blaxill, who reported all of this in their book, "If this wasn't a cover-up, it's hard to think of a polite synonym."

Although we can only speculate about the reason for their suspicious reporting, we know for a fact the CDC was well aware of the Thimerosal concern at that time. It was only six months later, in July 1999, that the American Academy of Pediatrics went around them to host a press conference asking for it to be phased out of use just in case.

Still, autism has been here forever, some claim now. Two new books this year have received great praise for their evidence to support that position. Autism has always been with us, they insist, people among us living in different tribes and different keys for centuries. And more importantly, it's great that it has. A little autism, one author suggests, is a helpful trait for humanity.

Further evidence of how the issue has evolved can be found in the title of the legislation first created to address the autism epidemic back in 2006. It was called The Combating Autism Act. As a nation, we needed to combat the condition with everything we had. Millions of dollars were allocated to determine how to handle it.

But by 2014, as the act got reauthorized, advocates of neurodiversity, the term used for those who want people to accept autism, not stop it, had convinced the government to change the name to The Autism CARES Act. I wrote a blog post called "The Autism Nobody Really Cares Act" in response. That's how it actually feels.

Mom and pop organizations born at the kitchen tables of parents of affected children, operating on a shoestring budget, were doing more to help families, prevent autism, give guidance, and make a meaningful difference than the millions of dollars the government had.

In ten years since its creation, the Interagency Autism Coordinating Committee has done nothing to help prevent, cure, or support a single case of autism that we are aware of. Our biggest fear is that it has only one agenda: find the supposed gene that causes it and use it to identify babies to abort. How's that for acceptance?

For those of us who live with the heartbreak and difficulty that autism presents, it's hard to capture the appropriate words to express the outrage we feel at these suggestions. They are not only dismissive of our children's needs, experiences, and challenges, they are arguably dangerous. Our society and our nation cannot sustain a population in which almost 4 percent of males have autism and may need lifelong services just to survive, as is the case now in New Jersey.

If autism has always been with us, isn't really that big of a deal, doesn't deserve to be treated, and it is offensive to do so, then we aren't dealing with the same disorder. There's been a major disconnect somewhere, and the type of thing they are describing is not the type of thing we are living. It is prudent that we immediately distinguish between the two possibly distinct forms of autism we seem to have, I believe.

This further undermines the credibility of the medical community, in my opinion. In all seriousness, they can't even get their story straight. It's genetic, but it's environmental. You're born with it, but you can regress. You can grow out of it, but it's permanent. You can have the features of it, but not have it. It's an avalanche, but it's always been here. On any given day, you can find a mainstream story with either position.

They can't have it all ways. They can't be the authority on autism and at the same time have no idea what autism is. They can't prop up population studies to rule out specific environmental factors when they can't even figure out what population has it.

No matter what they do, no matter how many people present with the disorder, no matter how many times they've been wrong throughout history, we're supposed to accept their position now. *Now* they know what they're talking about. *Now* they know how to diagnose it. Never mind the last seventy years when they didn't.

Furthermore, if they're going to make such a claim, they have to prove such a claim. They need to tease out, once and for all, the number of people diagnosed with Asperger's autism versus those diagnosed with Kanner's autism. They are not the same disorders. By muddying the waters, they are able to pull numbers out of thin air.

They also need to match the numbers of truly disabled adults we see on the waiting list in Florida, for example. In a *Dateline* special that aired in April 2015, it was shared that over 20,000 adults are anxiously awaiting to be taken care of for the rest of their lives. That's how disabled they are by their autism.

Now some people want us to believe this is how it has always been throughout humanity. Supposedly, we just didn't notice autism, write about it, hear about it, see it, treat it, house it, care for it, or describe it until 1943.

I personally find this speculation obnoxious. In every other area of my life, anyone trying to convince me I can't trust my own reality would be cause for panic and alarm.

We simply cannot allow for this, I believe. It's immoral.

Because the autism we have in our home, the autism my friends' children have, the autism I'm advocating for is not the autism that Einstein allegedly had. It's not the autism Jerry Seinfeld suggested he had (and then retracted with an apology . . . thank you, Jerry).

It's not the autism on *The Big Bang Theory*, either, the high-functioning, nerdy, brilliant caricature of autism that the world is happy to embrace. Once and for all—being a shy nerd who likes order and routine is not the equivalent of having autism.

The autism we had, that my friends' children have, that I finally started to see in my classroom around 2010, is not that kind of autism. These kids aren't getting married. They aren't working for NASA. They aren't sitting on federal advisory panels, capable of explaining how offended they are about anything. If you can be offended by this, you are not one of those I'm describing.

These are kids who, in their mildest form in my class, couldn't make a friend. Freaked out at the buzz of a light bulb. Had outbursts that frightened their classmates. Persevered on processes and procedures to their demise. Had almost zero social awareness.

These are kids who drove their teachers crazy, especially those older ones *who had never seen it before* and had no training in how to handle it. I had at least two teachers personally ask me to help them because they had no experience teaching students like these in their thirty plus years of teaching.

These are kids who might rock, and wear headphones, and like Elmo at the age of eighteen. Who have explosive diarrhea, life-threatening seizures, constipation, rage, self-injurious behaviors, and who wander away from loved ones and to water easily.

It's not called *Autism Goes to Medical School*, or *Autism Works for Google*, or *Autism Makes It to Age Forty-Five Without a Diagnosis*. It's called *Autism Speaks* for a very good reason. Most kids with autism can't!

Families are being crushed under the weight and the strain that their children's needs are putting on them emotionally, financially, and otherwise. So are schools, taxpayers, and emergency responders. To accept that, in my opinion, is to abandon the affected children . . . and for good reason. For many families, the serious issues autism may force them to face are anything but acceptable. In fact, many are quite horrific.

Chapter 14

Horror—Who Killed Alex Spourdalakis?

The short and technical answer to that question is his mother, Dorothy Spourdalakis. She admits to stabbing him to death before trying to take her own life in their suburban Chicago apartment in the summer of 2013, with the help of Alex's godmother, Jolanta Skordzka. Alex was a sixteen-year-old boy with severe, regressive, aggressive, nonverbal autism at the time.

The long answer to that question, however, examined in detail in the documentary by the same name, leaves you wondering who really was responsible. Was Alex truly the victim of a homicidal mother, eerily full circle as Bruno Bettelheim had once suggested, or were both he and Dorothy the victims of a medical community that had caused his autism, dismissed his autism, and had no idea how to treat his autism? The documentary makes a strong case for the latter. A jury will decide.

I was sitting in the parking lot of an elementary school when I got the news. While waiting for Emma to finish her special-education summer-school program that day, I stayed in my minivan listening to music. When I heard my phone buzz, I looked at the text with a gasp. "Alex is dead" is all it said.

Everything about it was horrific. From the way Alex had been initially handled at the hospital, left to wait in the emergency room for days, to the lack of ideas of how to help him, and even to the ignorance about what could be wrong with him to begin with, the whole thing had been a nightmare.

He was a nonverbal, large young man having physical outbursts; it was impossible to know what could be wrong. It was also scary. Alex had no way to communicate his pain other than to act out, a major concern of autism advocates for decades.

Imagine being in agony, perhaps with a migraine, a sore throat, acid reflux, a stomach ache, or even something like appendicitis, and having no way to communicate that to anyone.

Imagine being the parent of that child, watching them thrash around, scratch themselves, bite themselves, bang their heads against walls, tantrum, and scream incessantly while you play detective to figure it out. Imagine being accused of beating them or abusing them when you brought them to the hospital for help.

Imagine having a teenager in diapers with episodes of explosive diarrhea who isn't treated for it or taken seriously because they also have an autism diagnosis. Imagine being suspected of or investigated for abuse when you sought help because they didn't believe you that your child was self-injurious.

This is the reality of autism for many, unfortunately. Because it is still considered a psychiatric condition, co-morbid medical conditions, such as gastrointestinal distress, eczema, seizures, allergies, headaches, mitochondrial dysfunction, and so much more, aren't considered relevant. In fact, they are usually not even considered at all, wiped under the rug as just "part of the autism."

To date, autism does not have a standard of care. That means when a child with autism presents at a hospital or to a doctor, there is no medical practice in place for how to handle it. No blood work is officially ordered. No gastrointestinal work-ups are ordered. MRIs don't have to be done. Nothing actually has to be done, which is how Alex ended up sitting in the emergency room for several days. Literally, no one knew what to do with him.

Dorothy insisted that her son was suffering. As a mother with a child who also suffered from repeated infections, seizures, skin rashes, and more, I was inclined to believe her. I reached out to a friend I knew at the hospital to see what I could do. *Not much* was the answer.

In the hospital's defense, tests were run to see what they could find. They also looked for an outplacement for Alex, willing to transfer him, but those placements were psychiatric homes. Alex, his mother was adamant, did not need psychiatric help. He needed medical help.

A friend of mine had been in a similar situation a few years before. Her nonverbal teenaged son started punching himself in the face one day, thrashing around their home, and screaming in distress. It took several adults to strap him to a gurney and bring him to the hospital, where he remained restrained for his own safety. I wrote about it with her permission.

Eventually, it was confirmed that he was suffering from a serious bowel condition and was successfully treated; however, it was only because they had seen a specialist on the other side of the country who offered to look. Had she not had that resource, her son would have gone home with nothing being done to help him.

It's just another obstacle autism parents face, and very much a part of the reason it was determined that autism mothers show the same levels of stress on their brain scans as combat soldiers. Many autism parents are truly suffering from post-traumatic stress disorder. Only, to be fair, the "post-" should be eliminated. For some, the trauma never stops.

The number of medical doctors qualified and interested in caring for children on the spectrum, connecting the dots between their behavior and their physical well-being, is incredibly small. If autism is a psychiatric and permanent condition you are born with, learning to adapt to it and medicating it with psychotropic drugs would be the only way to go. Currently, for most doctors, it is.

And so Dorothy took Alex home after weeks of attempting to get help. In spite of the media coverage the story received while he was in the hospital, Alex's condition had not improved. It was then, she admitted in a suicide note, that she decided to kill him and herself.

The story divided the already very fractured autism community. The way the situation had been handled outraged many. Some believed Dorothy really was insane, in need of serious psychiatric help. Even if the stress of her son's condition had driven her to the brink, and even if the medical community were to blame for it, they argued, it didn't change the fact that Alex should have been removed from her care.

Others believed Dorothy was the ultimate victim of the medical community, driven to the brink, abandoned, and then labeled crazy. It was no better than Kanner or Bettelheim, they argued. Suggesting she was responsible was akin to betrayal.

However history records the story, the sad truth was this. Alex was dead. His mother, against all natural and maternal impulses, and according to her own admission, was responsible. And it wasn't the first time, or the last, it would happen. Just this year, a mother in Oregon got life in prison for tossing her six-year-old son with autism off a bridge.

As I looked around at the more than ten district buses lined up to take the one in eight children in special education home that day, I prayed it wouldn't happen to any of them.

Wandering—Avonte, Mason, and so many more

The most common way for children with autism to die is by wandering off. Claiming autism isn't deadly is a lie.

Nonverbal and severely affected children are most at risk, but it can happen to higher functioning children, too. Eloping, escaping, getting away from a caregiver, and even getting away from a school can happen to anyone. It's exactly what happened to Avonte Oquendo of New York.

On a normal school day one afternoon, fourteen-year-old Avonte slipped out the door with no one noticing. In spite of the fact that it was only a short period of time before his absence was confirmed, no more than eighteen minutes, it was too late. His remains washed up on the shore a few months later.

Many children died similarly before him. A five-year-old boy named Mason wandered only a short distance from his home and died in a nearby pond in 2010. Even my friend Michelle's daughter wandered away from a family party in her own backyard, drawn to the neighbor's pool, where she was found dead shortly thereafter.

The fear this stirs is hard to describe. On top of every other issue, autism parents have to be hyper-vigilant about their child's safety. I have friends that have bolted their doorways, boarded up windows, installed outrageously expensive alarm systems and fences, and have even gone so far as to sleep in front of their child's bedroom door at night. Some, like us, just move.

Even driving in a car isn't always safe. One mom I know has to keep her eight-year-old son in a car seat at all times. Without strapping him in such a way that he cannot undo it, he is inclined to open the doors while she's driving. One time, he almost succeeded.

To add to the stress, emergency responders have only been learning how to help in the last few years. Thanks in large part to the National Autism Association, their effort to supply families with devices that can track their children should they wander, coupled with their effort to educate emergency responders about how to handle autism, has helped improve the situation dramatically. In fact, they were instrumental in developing the diagnostic code a doctor can now add to a child's diagnosis for safety purposes.

But sadly, it hasn't been enough. So many families and emergency responders remain unequipped to handle the tsunami of children now affected by autism becoming adults. Stories of teenagers unable to respond to an officer's demands being arrested or even shot have been reported.

It raises questions that deserve answers. If autism has always been with us, where have all the stories of their wandering deaths been? How is it that the police haven't needed to be trained to deal with it until now?

Bullying: A bully on the bus

For a short period of time in second grade, I decided to drive Emma to and from school myself. A phone call from the school alerted me that some older kids were picking on her. I didn't ask why before deciding I didn't care. Emma was not taking that bus.

Like I had worried when I placed her on it at three years old, the bus was not a safe place, even though her bus driver was my neighbor, a lovely woman I trusted entirely. If keeping her safe meant I had to drive her back and forth, so be it.

Eventually, she begged to be let back on the bus, and reluctantly I gave it another try. Whether or not the bullying continued, I don't know. Although she could speak well by second grade, she had never mentioned it in the first place.

A friend of mine and managing editor of the *Age of Autism* blog, Kim Stagliano, was not so lucky on either account. Her child could not speak, and her bully was not a child; it was the bus driver. Cameras caught the driver taking her daughter's fingers and pulling them backward, twisting them, and hurting her. Only when Kim noticed a change in her daughter's behavior did she get suspicious. An investigation determined what had happened, and they won their case in court.

But she is not the only case. Multiple bus incidents and abusive drivers have been reported in the last few years, including cases when they have simply forgotten about a child they are transporting. When the nonverbal child can't speak up to alert that driver they haven't been dropped off, they get driven back to the bus barn to sit alone until they are found. Such was the 2015 case of nineteen-year-old Paul Lee, who had severe autism and was left on a hot bus for eight or nine hours. He died.

And then, of course, there are just the bullies, no bus needed. Perhaps no case better illustrates the danger children with autism may find themselves in from bullies than the case of a fifteen-year-old boy from Ohio. In 2014 he was lured to another teen's home on the premise he was participating in the ice-bucket challenge to raise awareness for ALS. When he got there, however, a bucket of feces and urine was dumped on his head.

Unsafe schools

As schools have been tasked with educating the tsunami of children on the spectrum and with other special needs, they, too, have been pushed to the brink. The cost of educating just one child with autism has been estimated at approximately $17,000 a year, approximately $8,600 of that paid for by the schools.

Multiply that by 1 in 68 students, the current rate of autism, and you can figure out pretty quickly how serious the situation is. A high school of two thousand students has approximately thirty students with autism to educate. That's $258,000 *a year* the school has to spend on autism alone.

Part of that expense is because many children with autism need a full-time aide. In our case, every aide Emma ever had has been a wonderful human being. It is the most important job to a special-needs parent, and yet it often gets paid the least. A caring, loving, competent aide is worth their weight in gold.

But not every child or parent gets one. Sadly, stories of poorly qualified, cruel, and downright abusive aides have been reported. Cameras have caught children being dragged down hallways, smacked across the face, yelled at, and put into isolation rooms for hours.

To be unsure that your child is safe in the hands of the people you are trusting to educate them is horrific. Thankfully, such situations are more an exception than the norm. Most educators care deeply for their students.

Still, I have long held the belief that once the education profession realizes it has been footing the bill for an epidemic that appears to have been caused by the medical profession, it will be the first to rise up and sue for damages. The amount of money the education profession, and the American taxpayer, have had to come up with to take care of these children is in the trillions.

Once people get that, and that we are in serious danger as a country, as the military has been warning for years that this generation of children is "Ready, Willing, and Unable to Serve" because they are so disabled, things may finally start to change.

Banishment and abandonment

Another serious concern for autism parents is long-term placement for their children. As the *Dateline* special in 2015 showcased, there simply aren't enough places for them to go when they become adults. Many friends of mine have joked they simply can't die as a result. There's actually nothing funny about what they are saying, though. They really can't.

According to the special, "Autism rates have more than doubled over the last decade . . . an estimated half a million young people will age out in the next ten years." "Aging out" is defined as being twenty-one years old. That is the last year a school district is legally obligated to educate a child.

As Linda Walder, the Executive Director of the Daniel Jordan Fiddle Foundation, an advocacy group for adults with autism, said in the report, "It's a tsunami of children who are aging to adult life. And we really have no safety net for them, or very few safety nets."

Her comments match a recent column published by *USA Today* in January 2016, "The coming avalanche of autistic adults." According to the column, there are over 1.5 million children with autism aged three to seventeen years old right now who will have virtually nowhere to go in the next decade or two if they need to move from home. This is arguably a public health crisis the likes of which we have never seen.

But even in cases where there will be some time before a long-term placement is needed, there have been incidents of neighbors taking autism families to court for just living next to them. Some children with autism are loud and have vocal tics and screaming fits that are difficult for others to live with. As heartless as it seems, it's happening. People don't want to live near autism families like that, and landlords don't want to rent to them. Where will they go?

Vulnerability and limitations

In our case, we are blessed that Emma has made such incredible progress that most people have no idea she was ever diagnosed unless they spend some real time with her. She's different, but she's not obviously disabled. Her disability is now primarily intellectual. Any physical manifestations of autism she used to have, such as rocking, hand flapping, and covering her ears, are long gone.

Even so, she's extremely vulnerable. She's just abled enough to seem fine, but just disabled enough not to be. Any charlatan who wants to sell her some magic beans will likely be successful.

And to what extent she'll ever be fully independent we're not sure. Abstract thought, including making change, is very difficult. For example, I found out this year that she isn't purchasing lunch at school on the days she doesn't bring one from home even though I have given her money. Without assistance, she is nervous to pay for things. She was embarrassed to ask for help or to tell me.

She is also painfully aware of how forgetful she can be. She overwhelmingly hates to be away from familiar places and people for fear of getting lost. Anytime we are somewhere new, she clings to my side, with rare exception. One time, she decided it was more important to take another turn on a carnival ride than stay by her brother, and we had to get the police involved to find her. Something like that has thankfully never happened since.

Additionally, the kind of job she'll have is realistically a low-level one. Emma isn't going to be a physics engineer like her brother or an astronaut like her younger sister plans. We don't even know if she'll be able to drive.

We will continue to do everything in our power to prepare her for independence, but we also have to be very mindful that she may never have it. Millions of parents wear these exact same shoes today.

Abuse: Dog cages, basements, and bed ties

There is a scene from a movie that has haunted me for years. In it, a child was kept in a hole in the ground in his parents' backyard. Afraid and unsure of what to do when he finds him, the main character does nothing.

That scene can be dismissed as fictional by many, but it hits very close to home in the autism community. Horror stories of desperate or despicable parents putting their children in cages, tying them to beds, or locking them in basements are not unheard of.

In 2013, a young boy was rescued from the cage where his parents had kept him. They claimed they had put him there for his own safety, as they didn't know how to handle him. In 2015, however, they were sentenced to seven years in jail for doing so.

There are other cases of abuse, much like the one previously described with the young man who had feces dumped on him.

Sexual abuse is also a serious threat for people with special needs, as they are three times more likely to be assaulted. Children with autism and intellectual disability are magnets for being taken advantage of.

Measuring the emotional and verbal abuse people with autism experience is harder to do. Even the best parents lose their tempers, pushed to the brink by the disorder and all of its demands. Sleep-deprived, isolated, afraid, and on the verge of a breakdown, plenty of parents have said things to their spouses and their affected children that they regret. I am one of them.

To be sure, not everything about having a child with autism is so horrific. Thankfully, for many, it's not. But to ignore these very real issues some autism families face on a daily basis, and worse, to suggest that they aren't real or something to be stressed over, is inhumane.

Frankly, anytime I hear someone suggest that they would rather have a child with autism than a dead child—their way of justifying autism as an acceptable vaccination outcome if it were true, as well as to dismiss the seriousness of the disorder and what it does to a child and a family—I have two immediate reactions.

One is to ask, brain damage or death? These are our choices? That's the safety standard we're willing to accept?

And two, to instantly dismiss them right back.

They have no idea what the hell they're talking about.

Chapter 15

Revolt—The Consequence of Coincidence

In August 2014, I logged on to my computer as I often do throughout the day. Scrolling through my newsfeed, I started to notice a pattern. A video with a fellow activist I knew, Dr. Brian Hooker, a scientific researcher and father of an affected child, had been created. Apparently he had found a whistleblower. The autism community was buzzing.

I watched the video intensely, not quite sure what to make of what I was hearing or seeing. On the other end of the phone call being recorded by Brian was the voice of a CDC scientist named Dr. William Thompson. I knew that name well.

Years before, after J. B. Handley put together a website to house the fourteen studies used to debunk a link between vaccines and autism, I asked him to write about them. As a layperson, I wanted to examine their findings, conflicts, and methodology. Other autism organizations and scientists had done most of that work already; really, I was just summarizing their critiques and looking for anything new that stood out to me.

I knew I recognized the name of William Thompson. I had all of the studies printed out in a binder I kept in my office. I pored over those studies, reading every word and taking notes. I knew them by name, year, and title. Dr. Thompson was the lead author of the 2007 *New England Journal of Medicine* study on Thimerosal and neurodevelopmental disorders.

This was the study that found a correlation between higher levels of mercury exposure with executive functioning and better fine motor skills, an outlandish conclusion that defies all common sense, in my opinion.

This was also the study Dr. Paul Offit and others used as the proverbial nail in the coffin in their argument that Thimerosal was safe and didn't hurt children. In an interview for the documentary film *Trace Amounts*, Dr. Offit claimed, "You had a definitive test, as far as I'm concerned, regarding Thimerosal safety. I mean, that study that Bill Thompson performed at the CDC in 2007 that was published in the *New England Journal of Medicine* was a wonderful study."

Well, maybe not. In the first place, they only looked at Thimerosal exposure through the first seven months of life, even though children could be vaccinated with it annually through a flu shot and other childhood vaccines beyond seven months. And as is always the case when using epidemiology to assess Thimerosal exposure outcomes, they *estimated* exposures. No one will ever know what each individual child actually got.

Additionally, the children most likely to be susceptible to Thimerosal were excluded from the study. Any children who had been diagnosed with encephalitis, meningitis, or hydrocephalus were excluded, as were low-birthweight babies, perhaps the most vulnerable children of all.

Worse, that study did not assess autism spectrum disorders. The very study being used to exonerate Thimerosal didn't even look at autism as an outcome. The study got rid of the children most likely to show a correlation before it even began.

And it was also the study that showed Thimerosal caused tics. It wasn't the first study to do so, either. David Kirby even wrote about it for the *Huffington Post* after it was published.

Dr. Thompson confirmed our concern about tics while speaking freely with Dr. Hooker, not knowing he was being recorded. Thimerosal causes tics, he claimed. He even acknowledged that tics were largely associated with autism, and we should start a campaign and make that our mantra.

Naively, after realizing the significance of what Dr. Hooker had shared and who had shared it with him, I thought the controversy would end. Dr. Thompson is not some low man on the totem pole at the CDC where autism research is concerned. He's among the top people involved.

It is extraordinary that he came forward of his own volition, making the effort to reach out to Dr. Hooker (Dr. Thompson called Dr. Hooker and not the other way around) and confess that he carried "great shame now when I meet with families with autism because I have been a part of the problem," as well as to admit that Thimerosal causes tics and he would never give a Thimerosal-containing vaccine to his own wife. (You can find the transcripts of their conversations in the book *Vaccine Whistleblower* by Kevin Barry.)

Equally extraordinary is the fact that he was willing to cooperate with Congress, turning over thousands of documents to verify his vaccine safety concerns. After retaining a lawyer from a firm specializing in federal whistleblower cases, he even issued a careful press release designed to reassure everyone that vaccines are safe and save lives, while at the same time acknowledging the CDC omitted important data from research on the MMR vaccine that could have validated Dr. Wakefield's hypothesis.

Dr. Thompson was a member of the CDC team that did the additional research Wakefield had called for. When they found statistically significant evidence that supported Dr. Wakefield, he claimed, they redid the study to make the link go away. He even discussed with Congressman William Posey, a Republican from Florida, how they got together to do it. On July 29, 2015, on the House Floor, Rep. Posey read a statement from Dr. William Thompson that described how they did it in detail. Most importantly, he acknowledged, "we intentionally withheld controversial findings from the final draft of the paper."

And so it seemed like the house of cards was finally going to fall. Although I hadn't quite exhaled, knowing anything in this controversy could happen, I felt confident that there was no way the CDC could back their way out of this one. The very man they relied on for the science to support their policies, program, and products had just confessed they were full of crap, and that he was ashamed of himself because of it.

But as the days went by and the press remained quiet, the internal knowing, the same voice that had been with me since Emma's birth, spoke up ever so softly. This wasn't going to do it either.

Somehow, some way, Bill Thompson was going to be twisted into a punch line, another cog in the conspiracy wheel, a man on the verge of a mental breakdown no one should take seriously. I even worried that if too much time passed, he would be pressured to change his story. We should trust his science, they would say, just not him.

Two more whistleblowers and a thief

In hindsight, I shouldn't have been that surprised. Two other whistleblowers had come forward before him with accusations of vaccine fraud. They were not CDC scientists; they worked for Merck. Stephen Krahling and Joan Wlochowski were virologists working on the MMR vaccine when Project 007 was implemented.

Named after the fictional spy, it was allegedly designed to hide the disturbing results of their findings. In short, the mumps component of the vaccine, they claim, isn't working well anymore. It may very well be the reason mumps outbreaks among college students have been popping up in recent years.

Krahling and Wlochowski decided to come forward with their concerns, and in 2010, they secured attorneys and brought a whistle-blower lawsuit forward. The case is still pending.

And lest we forget, there is also researcher Poul Thorsen. Thorsen is the original face of fraud in the autism controversy, a researcher from Denmark hired by the CDC as a part of the team looking at vaccines for their potential role in the autism epidemic.

Denmark was chosen as a good place to do research because of its system of socialized medicine and record keeping. The Danes had also lowered their use of Thimerosal in the early 1990s.

Thorsen was a part of the team to show Thimerosal may help prevent autism. When it was lowered in use there, the study claimed, autism rates skyrocketed. (A significant change in diagnostic procedures in Denmark that was very likely responsible for the illogical findings was omitted from the study.)

Thorsen is currently on the Department of Justice most-wanted list for allegedly embezzling over one million dollars of CDC funds for personal use. He is charged with thirteen counts of wire fraud and nine counts of money laundering. Even so, he remains a free man in Denmark today. Incredibly, it was recently discovered, the US government is still funding him.

Apparently it doesn't matter if you are accused of being a thief by the United States government when it comes to doing the most important research affecting the world's children. This is a man our CDC, and by default the IOM, has trusted to do the science to assure us vaccines don't cause autism.

Astroturf takes over

According to Emmy-award–winning journalist, former CBS National news correspondent, and author Sharyl Attkisson, *astroturf* is the name given to a modern phenomenon designed to control the public's perception of any given topic.

By portraying themselves as the majority, bloggers and commenters, often but not always anonymous and/or paid by industry, take over comment threads, Facebook posts, or Tweets to present their side of the story as the truth, as well as the one the majority of the public supports, even though that is usually untrue. In other words, they make it appear like they are the voice of the people, even though they usually are not: fake grass roots.

In her words,

> Astroturfers often disguise themselves and publish blogs, write letters to the editor, produce ads, start non-profits, establish Facebook and Twitter accounts, edit Wikipedia pages or simply post comments online to try to fool you into thinking an independent or grassroots movement is speaking.
>
> They use their partners in blogs and in the news media in an attempt to lend an air of legitimacy or impartiality to their efforts. Astroturf's biggest accomplishment is when it crosses over into semi-trusted news organizations that unquestioningly cite or copy it.

Sharyl identified her top ten "astroturfers" in 2016. Among them were several of the most widely recognized bloggers, authors, industry insiders, and commenters who attack "anti-vaxxers"; among them is Dr. Paul Offit.

For years, these people have criticized and bullied the vaccine safety movement, to put it mildly. Two examples came in 2014. The first was when they were able to convince national restaurant chain Chili's not to raise money for the National Autism Association's wandering prevention program; later, they convinced insurance company Allstate to revoke its deal with actor Rob Schneider for a commercial. Rob has been an outspoken critic of vaccine safety and government corruption.

Earlier, astroturfers also tried to go after Jenny McCarthy's position on the daytime talk show *The View*. In that instance, they were unsuccessful, an amazing show of strength on the part of ABC. Such public courage in the face of being accused of killing babies is rare. It's why so much of the support for vaccine-concerned parents remains behind the scenes.

For the worst thing a person, celebrity, politician, or business can be accused of these days is being "anti-vaccine," and astroturfers know it. No one wants to be a part of this controversy, or labeled that, let alone a huge corporation.

But by 2015, when everything would change with the outbreak of measles at Disneyland in California, astroturfing would elevate itself to a new level. It was no longer enough for them to go after people and organizations personally, professionally, and financially.

Now they were going after the very idea that anyone had the right to doubt the science and safety of vaccines at all. They were going after exemptions, the only real way you could assert your doubt. California was ground zero.

Mickey gets the measles

In the early fall of 2014, Eric Gladen approached me with a job offer. Eric was the guy I first met on the National Mall in Washington, DC, at the Green Our Vaccines Rally in 2008. He was the man who had been poisoned by Thimerosal at the age of twenty-nine after receiving a tetanus shot that contained it.

When he finally figured out what had happened to him and recovered, he dedicated his life to telling the story. He sold his home, bought an RV, and spent almost ten years making a movie about the experience. If a grown man could be poisoned by one shot, what could happen to a tiny baby repeatedly exposed to the chemical in the first few months of life? He decided to find out.

In 2014, the movie was finally ready. It was called *Trace Amounts,* in reference to the term used to describe the amount of Thimerosal still left in some vaccines. In my opinion, it was phenomenal. It was my life. We entered the controversy at the exact same time. Eric had thoroughly included everything I experienced in a decade.

More important to me was the fact that Eric could articulate what being poisoned with mercury felt like. Although his symptoms came on when he was an adult, and he never lost the ability to speak, he experienced much of what Emma would later describe. Hallucinations. Night terrors. Sensory impairment. Mood swings. ADHD. Eric was the living, breathing, surviving mouthpiece of what it felt like.

When he asked me to join his team as a consultant, I immediately accepted. I was in awe of what Eric had done, as well as deeply indebted. He created something that over the course of ninety minutes could explain in detail, and quite convincingly, what I had been dedicating myself to all this time.

Another person also believed in the movie. Robert F. Kennedy, Jr., who is quoted as saying he entered the vaccine controversy "kicking and screaming" back in the early 2000s, had not spoken out much by the end of the decade.

After watching the movie, however, he was inspired again to take up the fight. He never changed his position about what he believed happened, even more convinced that the powerful medical industrial complex, supported by a media that was dependent upon them financially and reluctant to report on them truthfully, had manipulated the science, covered up the truth, and orchestrated the worst fraud against the American people, perhaps ever. By far, he has been the most important weapon we parents have in our arsenal.

That fall, we worked hard to create a tour for the film. Eric and his co-director, Shiloh Levine, would travel the country to show the film in different locations from California to New York. A panel of experts would appear alongside them, from doctors, to politicians, to parents, and of course, RFK, Jr. He appeared at all of the major premieres.

The real premiere, however, the first time it would be screened anywhere, was at the Chinese Theater in Los Angeles on February 4, 2015. It had been secured to screen the film and present a panel discussion afterward. Several members of the media, along with several celebrities, joined us that evening. By all accounts it was very successful.

But in addition to the beautiful backdrop of the location, literally steps away from where the Oscars would be held only weeks later, we found ourselves amid a metaphoric backdrop of much larger importance. Only weeks before, the Ebola scare of 2014 had quickly morphed into something much less serious physically but much more serious politically.

There had been an outbreak of measles in California, allegedly beginning at Disneyland, the happiest place on earth. And its impact on our movie premiere, not to mention our country, our culture, and our liberty was about to go very viral, very quickly.

I believe the words you're looking for are "thank you"

Within weeks of the measles outbreak, the topic was hard to miss anywhere in the news. Although it involved fewer than 200 cases (in a country of over 350,000,000 people), you would have thought it was millions of children affected. And you would have thought that millions of children not only had the disease but were also dying from it.

The medical community was happy to present it this way, pointing their fingers with a shameful *tsk, tsk* at misinformed parents as the cause, and did nothing to calm people's fears. If anything, they capitalized on the outbreak, making measles seem significantly more deadly and dangerous than it actually is.

It was hard to ignore the craziness. Parents were being successfully pitted against other parents, a masterful manipulation. Once again, rather than examine why the medical community had lost the trust of a generation of parents, they got parents to turn on one another.

One father made his appearance on television with his child sick with cancer, claiming that the school should kick out any children not vaccinated to protect his. And one mother, upon learning her baby may have been exposed to the measles, lost her mind on a Facebook post that went viral. She was furious, absolutely furious, that she had to endure a week or so of fear of the measles.

By that point, I had had enough. There is only so much a parent can take. It wasn't bad enough that we parents had done "right" by society's standards when we followed doctors' orders to a T, and that we were being called liars, ignored medically, and wiped under the rug as irrelevant. Now we were being blamed for hurting other people's children by speaking out about the issue. I was done.

I put together my own Facebook post as an emotional plea for understanding and compassion. Within a few hours, it, too, took on a life of its own, and within a few days, it appeared on several blogs, one of which crashed from the traffic it was generating.

I based it on a post I had written almost a decade earlier when I tried to find the right analogy for the controversy. Many people have attempted to use car seats, drinking and driving, smoking, and seat belts as justification for mandatory vaccination. The enforcement of those laws, they argue, is proof that the government has the right to make you do something, or stop you from doing something, if it's for your own good and for the good of others.

But they are wrong. Those are not appropriate analogies. The enforcement of those laws cannot result in harm. Wearing a seat belt cannot hurt me. Wearing a helmet cannot hurt me. Not smoking if I like to smoke may be irritating, but it will not bring me physical harm.

Vaccines, however, carry inherent risk. They *can* kill you. They *can* cause brain damage. They *can* cause chronic disease. The only thing we are arguing about is how often it happens and to whom, thus the reason for the liability protection in the first place. The medical community, the pharmaceutical industry, and the government say it's rare. Consumers say it's not.

And so a more appropriate analogy for mandatory vaccines is the draft. We are literally in a war on infectious disease, and we have decided as a nation to put our children on the front lines of the defense; vaccines are the main weapon we are giving them to fight it.

Those of us who believed in the fight, supported the fight, and never questioned the worthiness of the fight, or our leaders, have learned the hard way that sometimes equipment backfires. Sometimes people die in wars from friendly fire. Sometimes things go terribly wrong, and the war they thought was worth fighting, in the end, really wasn't. The cost was too high.

But we have also learned something else, something that no child, no parent, and no family should ever have to learn like we did. That some children's deaths and injuries don't matter. That some children aren't worthy of being acknowledged. That rather than being heralded as heroes for their sacrifice, they are dismissed as acceptable collateral damage.

Under no circumstance are we to talk about our loss and scare others. The fact that most rewarded cases of vaccine injury are sealed, meaning if you want your money, you have to agree not to speak of it, proves it.

To reiterate, kids who die from vaccine-preventable diseases are victims that matter. Kids who die from vaccines designed to prevent those diseases are acceptable losses. This is how we think as a society and how we behave.

It would be bad enough if this is how we treated adults in any war. In fact, we saw the way the young men making their way back from Vietnam were treated and hopefully have learned from it. They didn't ask to be drafted either. They gave their lives to a questionable war and then were treated horribly for it by many. It was an embarrassing episode in our nation's history.

But so is this, even more so. These are our children! And when vaccines hurt them, the children deserve recognition, treatment, and respect. They deserve to be acknowledged, their names on a plaque equal to any other veteran in a war. And by God, they deserve the truth.

And this is why I believe we had the measles outbreak of 2015. Because a generation of parents put their children on the front lines only to find out the hard way *their kids don't matter*.

They also had to find out the hard way that the equipment was bad; that the armed services figured it out and hid it from them; that the very people responsible for allowing it to happen were also allowed to determine their own guilt, not to mention profit from it in the process; and that their damaged children wouldn't get acknowledgement or treatment anyway.

People have stopped believing in the war on infectious disease as they once had. The war against polio can hardly be considered equal to the war against chicken pox or hepatitis B, and yet they are treated the same. Likewise, they have stopped believing in the leaders that wage the war. The revolving door between policy makers and policy profiteers in the medical sector has made it impossible to trust their motives.

And they have stopped believing in the strategy used to fight it. Whistleblowers, alleged thieves, questionable science, political nonsense, fear mongering, attacking parents, astroturfing, sealed cases, manipulative legalese, shame, name-calling, threats, coercion, bullying, and pitting parents against parents have made the motive clear. It's not about protecting children. It's about protecting a profit, a product, and a program.

I wrote about all of this in a post called "I Believe the Words You're Looking for are Thank You." Rather than be scolded and attacked, I thought it was imperative to point out that many families had already lost a soldier in the war on infectious disease. A "thank you" would be more appropriate than the hate directed at them.

Furthermore, we acknowledged a long time ago as a society that there is only so much one family is supposed to give to any war. The movie *Saving Private Ryan* is a perfect example. That any mother should have to give up all of her children for any war is too much. Why would we ever expect a mother of a vaccine-injured child to vaccinate another child?

To be sure, it's not something this generation of mothers with injured children is willing to let happen without a fight. They'll be damned if they're going to be turned into the enemy now, too. Encouraging parents of enlisted soldiers to attack parents of fallen soldiers is as ugly as it gets.

My post changed a lot of minds. I had numerous people writing me privately to tell me they had never thought of it that way. Two months later, when I had dinner with a state senator, he told me the same thing. That analogy works because that analogy is right. We have betrayed the fallen soldiers and their families in the war on infectious disease, and we should be ashamed of ourselves.

Esai Morales, the famous actor, agreed. He shared my post on his Facebook page only a few days before I headed out to Los Angeles for the *Trace Amounts* premiere. I introduced myself to him that night as "the mom who wrote that post." Immediately, he called his wife over to meet me. She told me she cried her eyes out reading it.

Unfortunately, the movie couldn't withstand the heat from the measles controversy. Everywhere we went those few days, it followed us. My friends, the ones from the ballroom years before, were by my side, also working as consultants for the film.

One of their phones rang incessantly from reporters looking for an interview, including someone from a major news network. While sitting at a small table by our hotel, this news anchor admitted he was on our side but couldn't say it.

The whole experience was surreal. People have absolutely no idea how many people behind the scenes believe vaccines cause autism;

sometimes people in the very positions responsible for telling the world they don't.

Dr. Bill Thompson's quotes from the secretly recorded tapes had been incorporated into the movie. Eric did a wonderful job of making sure the audience understood the relevance and significance of these words.

Still, for the most part, he continued to be ignored. Not even a CDC whistleblower, the lead scientist on the 2007 *New England Journal of Medicine* study to exonerate Thimerosal, could get media attention.

The irony was mind-boggling. Here we were in the midst an outbreak of infectious disease being blamed on parents who had chosen not to vaccinate, many of whom at least in part had chosen not to vaccinate because they didn't trust the CDC, and the media wasn't the least bit interested in interviewing a whistleblower from the CDC who could validate their concerns. Heck, we couldn't even get most people to realize the whistleblower was real. It was devastating.

We walked down Hollywood Boulevard the day we were leaving in disgust and anger. The premier had been hijacked, the *LA Times* calling it an "anti-vaccine" movie, even though it was truly an anti-mercury and anti-corruption film.

On one side of the street stood Jimmy Kimmel's studio. He had just recorded a bit where doctors swore at the audience to "vaccinate your fucking kids." He, too, was misrepresenting the controversy, making fun of parents who had legitimate concerns, and picking on parents of vaccine-injured children. Once again, we were a punch line and a punching bag.

I walked over the star for Penn and Teller, who had also created a video to do something similar. I went back to it and stood on it for a few extra seconds just for the heck of it. The symbolism made me feel better, even though it was only for a moment.

Later that day, I flew home to a freezing Chicagoland. Although I missed the warm temperatures of Southern California, it wouldn't be long before I found myself back in the heat of things. Democrats across the country were about to use the measles mania to their advantage. Exemptions everywhere they were in control were about to disappear.

Chapter 16

Testimony—Let the Science, and the Mothers, Speak

As the measles hysteria grew, the medical industrial complex took the opportunity to go after exemptions. Throughout the previous decade, as worried parents began opting out of the vaccine program by the thousands, the leaders of the medical community had been waiting for the right disease to show parents how irresponsible they were to make that choice, as well as to get rid of the laws that allowed them to do so in the first place: exemptions. The measles outbreak was the perfect backdrop to go on the offensive.

Depending on which state you live in, people have the right to various vaccine exemptions. In some states, citizens have tremendous liberty to choose to vaccinate or not by using a personal belief exemption. In most states, however, you only have the option of religious and/or medical exemptions. By 2015, regardless of what options existed, the number of parents who were exercising their right to use them was increasing.

After the measles mania, the gloves were officially off. If the medical community couldn't get parents to trust them by publishing their own safety studies, demonizing parents who didn't trust them, banishing parents from their practices, and censoring the media, they were willing to go to the next level.

You simply wouldn't have the choice but to do what they said. By law, you were going to do what you were told whether you liked it or not. If that meant taking all exemptions away, so be it.

By spring, the effort to get rid of exemptions started sweeping the nation. It also quickly became partisan. Blue folks tend to believe public health trumps personal liberty and informed consent. Red folks tend to believe liberty and informed consent trump public health. As such, the move to get rid of all personal, religious, and even in some cases medical, exemptions to vaccines typically began in states where the Democrats had control. California and Illinois were among the first.

Prominent Democrats began speaking out in support of forced vaccination, urging lawmakers and leaders to protect children from irresponsible parents. Hillary Clinton even went so far as to publish a Tweet in support, equating questioning the efficacy of vaccines with not believing the Earth is round.

It was a perfect example of the condescension aimed at vaccine-hesitant parents. Questioning vaccine safety was akin to being a flat-Earther, they claim. (I've always found it odd they use that analogy. We are the ones telling everyone the earth is round, not the other way around.)

But as I thought about what she said, I had to give her props for being so politically savvy. Hardly anyone was questioning whether vaccines *worked.* Although a group of truly anti-vaccine people had formed and become more public by then, the majority of people concerned about vaccine safety, filing exemptions, and selectively vaccinating were not against all vaccines. It was the program, the policies, and the policy makers they didn't trust.

Thankfully, not all Democrats were as smug as Hillary or Dr. Richard Pan, a state senator and pediatrician in California, the man most responsible for the loss of exemptions there by the end of the summer. At least one Democrat was speaking out against the power grab of an agency and an industry that had been repeatedly found by government investigations to be corrupt.

"A cesspool of corruption" is, in fact, what the CDC had been called by one of the most famous Democrats in our country. Under no circumstances were citizens to give up any more of their rights to an agency or an industry that couldn't be trusted, especially if it had an impact on their children. Robert F. Kennedy, Jr., was determined to make sure of it.

A dinner for the Democrats

By the end of February, as predicted, Illinois unleashed a bill to tighten its exemptions. Unlike California, Illinois didn't have a personal belief exemption, only religious and medical ones. Although the medical exemptions weren't easy to get, securing a religious one wasn't very difficult.

The new bill wanted to make it much harder. If you were going to claim a religious exemption, a religious leader would have to sign off on your form and notarize it. Additionally, you would have to sit down with a doctor, every year, and learn about all of the reasons you were making a bad decision.

You simply needed to be educated, they believed, talked to about why you were misinformed and misled. And if that didn't work, you would have to sign a form that basically said you are a bad human being, a bad parent, and an irresponsible, selfish asshole that doesn't mind putting other people, including children, in jeopardy.

To put it mildly, we objected. That any parent needed to prove why we couldn't trust the CDC or the pharmaceutical industry was laughable. But it was real. They were serious, and we needed to act.

A friend of mine named Laura, an autism mother who lives in the state's capital and is a former lobbyist, has been instrumental in getting anything done politically in Illinois regarding autism since the early 2000s. Laura was responsible for the legislation that established a statewide program for early diagnosis. She was also responsible for the Mercury Free Vaccine Act, which, although intended to prevent the usage of any mercury-containing vaccine in Illinois, has been repeatedly circumvented by the Department of Public Health for various reasons.

She is incredibly smart and incredibly well connected. She knows the legislators, the language, and the game.

We spoke at length about what to do. The writing on the wall seemed fairly obvious. Illinois, the home of President Obama, was as blue as it got. Even though a very conservative Republican, Bruce Rauner, had been elected governor the year before, there was no way we could stop this bill.

At best, we could modify it. If we could expand the ability to get medical exemptions, which was truly what most people wanted anyway, and the most we could hope for, it was something. We might also be able to modify the rules for getting a religious exemption to be not quite as draconian.

To help make our case, we came up with an idea. We could use Bobby Kennedy to our advantage. By having him testify to the Senate on the bill, coupled with showing the legislators *Trace Amounts* and having a nice dinner with them to speak with them personally, perhaps we could change their minds. The Kennedy name still carries a lot of weight, especially among Illinois Democrats. Maybe they would listen to him.

After we reached out to Bobby and Eric, they agreed to make the trip. My friend and I quickly secured a movie theater, a restaurant, and created invitations to the event. Several senators confirmed their interest and commitment to the evening. But first, we asked they joined us in the Senate that afternoon for Bobby's testimony.

He was incredible. He eloquently laid out the case against making any changes to getting vaccine exemptions to a packed room. Until the CDC could clean up their act, he implored, making it more difficult for parents to opt out was a mistake.

I tried to take notes as I sat in the row behind him. I had heard him speak at the rally in 2008, on various talk shows, and before and after the movie premiere in February. But this was different. Here in the halls of the Capitol Building, he was completely at ease, the legacy of his name on full display for all to see. He was magnificent.

Afterward, we walked together throughout the building. In the hallway, there was a news crew waiting to interview him. People everywhere, after recognizing who he was, asked to come and take pictures.

Every so often, it would dawn on me whom I was driving around in my minivan filled with my kids' crap, stains from who knows what and who knows when, and a bag of soccer stuff in the back. I cringed at the memory of asking him something while he rode next to me in the front seat, probably one of the most awkward moments of my life.

"Um . . . Mr. Kennedy? I'm sorry, but that beeping means you have to put your seat belt on."

My God. I had just asked the nephew of one of our most beloved presidents, the son of an equally beloved senator, and basically American royalty, to buckle up. What in the hell had happened to my life?

By the time our dinner and movie rolled around, we were exhausted. I had chosen the wrong shoes that day, a pair of dressy black heels that were too tight. When we realized we left Bobby's book *Thimerosal: Let the Science Speak*, a meta-analysis of all of the biological science ever done on Thimerosal, in my friend's car, I got chosen to run outside and get it. Bobby was adamant that legislators learn the truth about the toxicity of Thimerosal before they ruled. I was in tremendous pain and full of blisters as a result.

It was just another thing to laugh about as we finally got a glass of wine and waited for the Democrats to arrive to our private dinner. We were cracking up. If you can't laugh at this life, you can't survive.

My friend had done a face plant outside of the building right in front of Bobby. Mortified, she needed his help to get up.

And then there was the elevator experience. When it opened for us to step in, a sea of yellow-shirted, pro-gun, Tea Party supporters were inside. A Kennedy standing in the middle of them was a sight to behold. You should have seen their faces, and later mine, as one of them came up to me while I was talking with Bobby an hour later in the hall.

"Hey, aren't you Julie?" A sweet older woman with gun buttons and a yellow shirt approached. She recognized me from an event I had just been to. I was running for school board back at home and got asked to speak by some Republicans.

"It's so nice to see you again!" she said sincerely. "What are you doing here?"

After I explained, she and her friend complimented me on taking up the fight.

"We didn't know a single person with autism growing up," they nodded in agreement to one another.

"Yeah," said the woman who had recognized me. "I had never even heard of it until my grandniece was diagnosed a few years ago."

That night, the dinner felt like a success. I sat at the table with Bobby and at least four other state senators for the meal, the only nonpolitical figure there. Everyone was kind, funny, and wonderful. We talked like old friends, discussing everything from our favorite television shows to Bobby's time in prison in Puerto Rico. I hadn't known he was fluent in Spanish like me.

I had not expected to sit among them for dinner when one of the senators invited me to do so. I was also not expecting the only female senator to join us that night to offer to take me shopping next door for shoes because my feet hurt so badly. Naively, I thought her kindness meant we had changed her mind.

Let this mother speak

When the bill finally came to a vote in the Senate committee, I made another trip down to Springfield. The only thing we could do at that point was speak from the heart and try to convince any Democrats on the fence that this wasn't a battle about anyone's faith in God; it was about their faith in organized medicine.

We were supposed to be heard at 2 p.m., but a fight over the budget put the hearing behind. For hours we sat in the hallway outside the room in which the vote on the bill would take place, surrounded by lobbyists for the medical community and a bunch of medical students in white coats. It was uncomfortable to say the least.

At one point, a female lobbyist for the other side came over and introduced herself to me sitting on the bench. She had her children with her, both older, and she explained that she wanted them to experience this.

She also asked me if I was my friend, the woman responsible for us having any dog in the fight at all. She needed to apologize, she claimed. She felt badly for how she had treated her on an email thread.

It solidified for me what I had known for some time. People just do not behave the same way behind a computer screen that they do face to face. Here, next to me, she was just another mom, a woman who felt as passionately about her cause, vaccination, as I did about mine, corruption.

We talked about our positions, and she acknowledged I had a point. She agreed medically fragile children should not be held to the same mandates as healthy children, and she even agreed their siblings shouldn't either. When I told her all moms have their children's best interests at heart, she put her hand on my shoulder and nodded.

Why anyone felt it was so urgent to make exemptions harder for those families with vulnerable children was beyond me, I continued.

In Illinois, even though exemptions had gone up, vaccine compliance rates were still over 95 percent.

"Well, we've had this bill in the works for over two years," she explained. "We've just been waiting for the right time to drop it."

"And the measles was the right time?" I questioned carefully.

"Oh yeah," she laughed. "Perfect."

If there had been any doubt, it was now gone. Those in the medical industrial complex knew exactly what they were doing.

In the room, we sat on opposite sides. Behind us the rows were filled with white coats and lobbyists to support the public health department. Several of the Democrats on the panel were the very people we had spent the evening with when Bobby came. Unlike then, I noticed, they were no longer warm and friendly. My friend and I could barely get them to make eye contact.

After those in favor of the bill had a chance to testify, my friend was given her chance. She started to tell her story, but quickly got cut off by one of the senators, who clearly wasn't interested in what she had to say. Thinking quickly, my friend asked if I could speak instead.

"I have a mother with me who has traveled almost four hours to be here today to speak to you. Can she please?"

"She has five minutes," the female senator who offered to take me shoe shopping stated coldly.

I got up and scooted to the microphone, also irritated. I couldn't find the speech I wrote at home and had to rely on my memory. As fast as I could, I tried to frame the issue for what it was, a crisis of faith in preventative medicine, not a religious crisis. This lack of faith resulted in increasing exemptions, which was why there was now interest in making these exemptions harder to get. I warned the senators that this problem wasn't going to go away until the crisis of faith in our public health agencies was resolved. It would only get worse.

I made a comparison to education, stating that if the teaching profession had 52 percent of their population of students failing (the current rate of chronic disease among American children, including obesity), it's unlikely that we could pass a law stipulating that no one could get out of a having a public education. Why was it that teachers were always fully accountable for the health of their students' education, but doctors weren't at all accountable for the health of their patients' bodies?

No one, except a child's parents, has more of an influence on their health than their doctor. Despite being the most vaccinated children in the world, our children are also the sickest. We have the most chronically ill children in the world. And, according to the 2016 estimate of the CDC, one in seven American children has a disability. One in seven.

Something is wrong. What they're doing isn't working. Parents can see that, so they are in for a fight for years to come, I warned.

I made several more compelling points, but in the end, it didn't matter. Although I did change one Democrat's mind, she changed her vote back to support the bill after getting a stern look from the committee leader. The vote was 6 to 3, Democrats to Republicans. Mandated vaccination was officially a partisan issue.

Miguel Jara

Around that time, a friend sent me an article from Spain. Her cousin was living there and shared a link to an article by a journalist, Miguel Jara, that she thought I'd find interesting. Miguel is an investigative journalist who writes about health issues in Spain, primarily regarding vaccines and medications.

He and his colleague, an attorney, assist families negatively affected by both. Currently, they are helping families go after damages caused by the Gardasil vaccine. Around the world, this vaccine is receiving tremendous negative attention for the harm it is causing. Spain is no exception.

Miguel was reporting on other vaccine issues as well. It turned out he had written a book on vaccines. I read his blog in detail and decided to reach out to him. I also ordered his book.

I had a number of questions. For years, I heard that other countries didn't vaccinate nearly as aggressively as we do, but I hadn't been able to verify what the schedules and policies were internationally. For the first time, I could ask someone directly. I wanted to know, what does vaccination look like in Spain?

Miguel responded right away. To my surprise, it was significantly different from here. In Spain, vaccination is *completely voluntary*. Spaniards do not believe the government has the right to force anyone to vaccinate, no matter the infectious disease.

I was stunned. I had heard that other countries were more relaxed with their policies, but I had assumed all first-world nations enforced mandatory vaccination to some extent. Not the case, Miguel reiterated. And not only that, they presented their options for vaccinating very differently than we did.

In Spain, vaccinations are placed into categories based on a risk–reward ratio: highly recommended, recommended, or personally recommended. A highly recommended vaccine would be for a highly contagious, very deadly disease. Recommended vaccines would include those for uncomfortable, contagious, annoying, but hardly-ever-deadly diseases. And personally recommended vaccines reflected travel needs, age, occupation, and lifestyle choices.

Most interestingly, and contrary to everything I had heard for a decade here in the United States, over 95 percent of Spaniards were still vaccinated against diseases in the highly recommended vaccine category despite the fact they had the choice not to be. People, it turns out, actually don't want to die from deadly infectious disease.

But nor do they want to be a continuous profit source for the pharmaceutical industry. Spain also doesn't allow advertising from the pharmaceutical industry. The trust between patients and doctors is extremely high, Miguel claimed.

It was so logical and so reasonable. It was exactly what we needed to do here in the United States, and fast. I wrote about our conversation with Miguel's permission for *Age of Autism*. Contrary to how the controversy gets presented, no one wants to die from an infectious disease. No one wants to put anyone else in harm's way, either.

But no one wants to be manipulated or mandated into taking an unnecessary risk with his or her life with no ability to hold anyone accountable if something happens. No one wants to be acceptable collateral damage, dead or disabled with chronic disease in the name of prevention. Brain damage or death is an unacceptable standard for safety.

Spain agrees. Drug companies do not have liability protection there. Television shows like *Law and Order* and *Chicago Med* aren't produced to shame non-vaccinating families into believing they are the devil or to convince everyone that all it takes is one child to destroy the world for everyone.

Millions of people have chosen not to vaccinate or "selectively" vaccinate in Spain, which happens to be the only way you actually can vaccinate there anyway. Amazingly, no one seems to care.

I have a job offer for you

In May, I met with Eric at a restaurant in Chicago. Like the year before, he had something to ask me. Was I interested in working for Bobby?

At first, I laughed. I thought he was kidding. My name had come up as someone who could be helpful as an assistant to him. Although he had an amazing personal assistant already, he was interested in working with someone who would be able to help him with the vaccine controversy exclusively. I was one of the choices.

I was flattered, but I immediately turned it down. I remembered what it was like in Springfield that day with him, watching how fast-paced and stressful his life was. He was a machine, clearly conditioned his whole life to handle politicians and politics.

When he said jump, people said, how high? Even an Eli Lilly lobbyist had gone to get him a soda while we were there, maybe one of the most ironic things I have ever seen in my life. (Bobby had no idea who she was. We only knew because my friend recognized her.)

Crazier, his cousin Caroline had been issued a death threat that day in Japan. It was on the news while we were in a senator's office. When we acknowledged it and expressed sympathy, he simply said, "We always have death threats in our family." And that was that.

I was in no position to handle that, I told Eric. My personal life was falling apart as we spoke. I had no idea what was going to happen, nor did I think I could be of any help. Thanks, but no thanks.

A friend told me to think about it. She wants me to run for office someday, and she thought this would be an incredible opportunity. I also told her to forget it, but it was too late. She planted a seed. By the end of July, I accepted the job.

Trace Amounts made some headway that summer. With all of the controversy in California over exemptions, it found its way onto the screens of several celebrities who Tweeted about it. Cindy Crawford, Ricky Lake, Alicia Silverstone, Ed Begley, Jr., and several others found the courage to promote it.

So did Jim Carrey. Out of the blue, he was back on the stage of vaccine safety. As he told us at a private meeting later that summer, he joked that he "came out of the box a little hot." The *Huffington Post* was immediately all over him about being anti-vaccine.

In August, in one of the most incredible experiences of my life, I traveled with Bobby to the United Nations, where *Trace Amounts* was shown to an audience as a part of an environmental conference. Later that night, we raised money for the cause on a magnificent yacht cruise down the Hudson River.

Hearings and rulings

Several important rulings have attempted to quash the vaccine debate once and for all. In 2009, the vaccine court, ruling on the omnibus decision of 5,000 families claiming vaccines had caused their child's autism (and pulling out Hannah Poling to compensate her on the side), had made it very clear vaccines had nothing to do with it.

In fact, one special master went out of her way to dismiss the connection between vaccines and autism, going so far as to claim you'd have ". . . to believe six things before breakfast" to think it did. It always struck me as ironic she chose a line from *Alice in Wonderland*, the most famous story of mercury poisoning in the world, as the way to say vaccines with mercury could not cause the symptoms of mercury poisoning in a child that had been vaccinated with mercury . . . and you were crazy to think they could.

It will be interesting to see how things play out with William Thompson, too, if they ever do. For if the CDC manipulated the science to exonerate vaccines, and that science is what was used to throw out those cases, then they are very possibly guilty of obstructing justice. In so many ways, all hell will break loose.

Then again, maybe not. In 2011, there was another important ruling. The parents of Hannah Bruesewitz took their case against Wyeth all the way to the Supreme Court. They wanted to be able to sue the pharmaceutical company directly for her injuries due to a vaccine that was eventually taken off the market, but the Supreme Court ruled against them. The late Justice Scalia wrote the deciding opinion.

Similarly, Congressional hearings about the subject have done little to help. Since the year 2000, several hearings about corruption, conflicts of interest, sketchy science, and more have been held without doing much to effect any meaningful change.

And although Representative Jason Chaffetz, a Republican from Utah and the current leader of the Government Oversight and Reform Committee, originally stated he would hold hearings on Dr. William Thompson, he has since changed his mind. Even the White House has dismissed the Thompson story as conspiracy theory.

So it's not without reason parents of vaccine-injured children are feeling mostly defeated and dismissed. Over and over again, the powers that be have ruled that their children actually weren't injured and that, even if they were, it doesn't matter. There was nothing that could have been done or should have been done to prevent it. Furthermore, suggesting otherwise and opting out of the program just in case selfishly jeopardizes public health. Shut up and do your duty, they have asserted. Everything is fine.

For one father, however, everything is still not fine. The vaccine court dismissed his son's severe and debilitating autism after a vaccine reaction as coincidental, but he isn't buying it. Unlike most parents in the omnibus, he is an attorney, and he is exercising his right to take the case to a traditional court now.

Bobby Kennedy has agreed to help him. In early 2016, he made his way to the courtroom to do the opening arguments. After a powerful objection, the doctors being sued for malpractice lost their request to have the case dismissed.

The judge wants to hear the case. And he wants Dr. William Thompson deposed in the process. So does Representative Mark Meadows, a Republican from North Carolina. He wants to hold a Congressional hearing.

Bent, not broken

We sat a few feet apart from one another at the little table in the waiting room, but we couldn't have been more distant otherwise. For the second time in three years, we had separated, the same issues still plaguing our fragile marriage. Love, it had begun to seem, was simply not going to be enough.

When it came to our daughter, however, we were still a united front. The previous summer, while having a wonderful day at the lake house, Emma had bent over in her swimsuit to pick something up. The left side of her back had a hump when she did.

Horrified, I ran my fingers over her spine. I couldn't tell if what I was feeling was muscular or skeletal but was more inclined to believe the former. Emma had always been weaker on her right side, ever since she was a toddler. It had been documented in her gigantic file.

And so I tried not to panic. Instead, I decided, I would place a call to one of my relatives who had a thriving chiropractic practice. We had taken a few years off from therapies, diets, and other interventions around the age of twelve.

I assumed she had simply grown weaker without therapy. All of the guilt I thought I had successfully put behind me came flooding back. Perhaps if we had kept up with physical and occupational therapy for these few years, this wouldn't have happened. We would never know.

Within a few days, I had an appointment to see a local chiropractor. He had worked with Emma five years earlier and still had her x-rays on file. When he showed me the new ones, I almost cried.

Emma's spine now looked like a snake. The normal curves from the first pictures had morphed into a gigantic "s." I was shocked, as she had had a school physical about a year and a half before that showed no evidence of a serious problem.

The fact that you could hardly see anything wrong with her from the outside seemed astounding, but then again, that's how everything wrong with Emma always was. That she never complained about it, went about her life normally, and didn't look like anything was plaguing her was hard to believe. When people looked at the images of her spine, they gasped.

For a few months, we tried chiropractic care. It was a long shot, but if it could work without having to do surgery, I was willing to try it. Several days a week we would head to the practice to get her adjusted. When it didn't seem to be working, at least partly because of the fact that we just couldn't go as often as they wanted, I decided we needed another opinion.

It turned out that one of the leading scoliosis surgeons in the world had an office about two miles from our home. He travels the world four times a year to do the surgery in impoverished nations for needy children. I instantly knew he was the person to trust with her care, and by Christmas, he confirmed she qualified for surgery.

It was good news, he explained, not at all making light of the seriousness of the problem. Because her curves were bad enough, there was no question about whether or not to brace her spine for two years; it wasn't an option. Additionally, there would be no problem getting our insurance to cover it. It more than qualified for the procedure.

We agreed to go the surgical route, aiming to schedule it for the next summer. They would cut her open from the bottom of her neck all the way to her lower back, drill nineteen screws into various spinal bones, and insert two rods to realign her spine when they were done.

She would need a three- to four-day hospital stay and several weeks at home to recover. All in all, we were looking at about a month of discomfort. He insisted she would be good as new after that.

And so here we sat, Mike and I, on a hot day at the end of July, both of us on our computers, headphones in, barely speaking, waiting as the hours ticked by. I should have been out of my mind with worry, but I was not.

Besides the heartbreak I felt about my marriage, I was almost completely at peace. Almost, I say, because I was somewhat conflicted by the outpouring of support we were receiving from everyone.

It sounds ridiculous, I know. Of course I was humbled and grateful for their love, prayers, and concerns. It just reminded me of how much people still misunderstood the trauma and seriousness of regressive autism.

Ten years on, organized medicine still doesn't believe it's real. And the movements to normalize it, accept it, and embrace it as a quirky gift that means you are a genius are making it even harder for people to understand.

This surgery, although admittedly very serious and very painful, was *nothing* compared to regressive autism. It was nothing compared to what she and we had been through. If anything, it felt like a walk in the park.

At no point in time did I have to argue with anyone over what was wrong with her. At no point in time did I get blamed for it. No one doubted what had happened to her, questioned me, or flat out accused me of lying about it. No one told me she always had it but that I just didn't remember that she did.

No one criticized me for getting medical treatment, accusing me of not loving her for who she is because of it. Not one insurance claim was challenged. The nurses and doctors were always wonderful, kind, and considerate, constantly checking on her and us. I didn't get scolded or shamed by them once.

I didn't have to learn about scoliosis, setting up a makeshift library in the dining room, downloading studies from the Internet, and getting medical textbooks to study its origin, its treatment, or any of the advancements in surgery over the years. There was no controversy surrounding it.

I didn't have to go on a waiting list for months to get a doctor to diagnose or treat her, or fly around the country to find someone who could. I didn't get asked to leave this doctor's practice for asking questions or challenging him.

I wasn't worried about talking about it with anyone; I was free to share our experience without wondering if that person now believed I was a conspiracy-theory nutjob. People had no idea how much I actually hated talking about autism, especially with anyone I had just met, for that very reason.

With scoliosis, I didn't have to choose my words carefully, constantly apologize and explain myself, or compare myself to the other mothers in the room.

Why Emma? Why me? Why not them?

Those thoughts didn't occur to me as I sat checking my email and updating my status while we waited for her to come out of surgery. Instead, I thought about the medical reasons she was still in there.

I had once asked the doctor why he believed Emma had scoliosis, curious if it had anything to do with her history. It may or may not, I reasoned. It runs in our family. Her great grandmother had a slight case, and so do I.

He didn't know for sure, he told us honestly. There were two kinds of scoliosis he was used to seeing. Idiopathic, the kind that just came on out of the blue with no known cause or origin, and neurologically caused scoliosis, the kind that came on after a brain injury in infancy.

He showed me pictures of children with cerebral palsy who suffered from the condition terribly. A lack of oxygen to their brain had had an impact on the development of their skeletal system.

I asked if children with mitochondrial disorders who also had trouble utilizing oxygen properly, those with low muscle tone, or even those with a toxic encephalopathy could have the same result.

They could, he confirmed; absolutely they could. And in that moment, I knew: there was probably nothing idiopathic about Emma's scoliosis whatsoever.

She recovered wonderfully from the surgery, just like the doctor had said she would. In less than a month, she started her first day of high school as if nothing had happened to her. The doctor insisted she had nothing to worry about, either. With her new back, she was stronger than ever.

We, too, recovered months later. We joke that we also needed surgery to finally correct the skeleton of our marriage, realign our priorities and our lives, and reinforce the commitment we had to one another and our family. We are trying to be stronger than ever, too.

In the end, autism bent us all in so many ways, but it did not break us.

EPILOGUE

Today, Emma is a happy, substantially healthier, fifteen-year-old girl. While she is still socially immature and sometimes needs prompting to switch from one activity to the next without resistance, she is fully verbal, has no sensory input problems, no obsessive interests or patterns, is able to independently care for herself, and lives a full, normal life. She is in Girl Scouts, Best Buddies, and is on the high school bowling team.

Beautifully, she also has friends. She likes to spend her time talking with them via Skype on the computer, playing three-dimensional spatial games like Minecraft. According to all of her testing, it is the one area in which she tests superior. Her ability to see a whole picture, design a room, and be creative is remarkable. She is also quite the artist.

Most importantly, she is quite the caring kid. While she can be stubborn sometimes, and she can still be hard to reach at times, she is often very thoughtful, very considerate, and very loving. As an example, she recently got upset when I wouldn't let her order $1,000 worth of sweatshirts she designed for thirty classmates to wear with her on St. Patrick's Day.

In most ways, we lead a very normal life. We take vacations, have dinner together, go to church, and have conversations, and we do so without incident, supervision, meltdowns, or worrying about anyone's safety.

But in so many ways, we lead an abnormal life as well. We are a family who appears to have it all together, but who has imploded more than once. We are a family who seems to have gotten through the worst, but who will likely have to take legal guardianship of their child in a few years for her own physical and financial safety.

We are a family who believes so deeply in the miracles of modern medicine that we help raise and donate tens of thousands of dollars a year so children on the spectrum can have access to it, but who are simultaneously despised by modern medicine for criticizing the harm it can cause.

We are a family who vaccinated, and yet are called "anti-vaxxers."

I got physically sick after writing this memoir. For two weeks, I couldn't sleep, had an upset stomach, and felt just as badly as I did on the basement floor. Revisiting the trauma of the early years, thinking I had put it all behind me, and opening up those old wounds was not something I wanted to do. All of the guilt, all of the pain, all of things I wish I could have done over again came flooding back. God, the guilt.

Mostly, I worried about judgment. No one knows the mistakes I made better than I. The number of nights I have lost sleep wishing I could go back in time to listen to my gut and call the doctor about my concerns and my fish consumption is countless. Even so, I'm no longer convinced I would have been told anything other than that she was fine and that everything I did back then was safe.

In fact, horrifically, in June 2014, the FDA updated their advice to encourage pregnant women, breastfeeding mothers, and children to eat *more* fish. They now advise them to eat *at least* two to three cans of light canned tuna, salmon, shrimp, tilapia, catfish, and cod per week. According to this change, I did exactly what I was supposed to when I was breastfeeding Emma. In fact, they claim, I actually should have been eating even more.

Unfortunately, I believe this is horrible advice, another link in the long chain of mercury tragedies we won't identify until it's too late. This advice pays no mind to the existing body burden of mercury women already have; to the synergy mercury has with hormones, antibiotics, and other medicines and toxins; or to the genetic vulnerability of each individual.

We must do more to bring awareness of the dangers of mercury to mankind. We must do more to protect ourselves. We will continue suffering tragedies, as we have throughout history, until we finally learn our lesson. We have much to learn.

But, I constantly have to remind myself, I was not that mom. I was not the mom we always see in the movies, confidently yelling at the doctors, telling them how to do their job, or making a scene.

No, I was the quiet, obedient mom who did what she was told and who believed what she was told, even when she could feel it was wrong. I was the mom that put other people's opinions over her own instinct.

I sobbed one afternoon, about to call my publisher to table the book. Why in the world would I want to open my life like this? Why would I subject myself to this? I cried to my husband. I can already predict the criticism . . . *anti-vaccine, conspiracy-theory mom perpetuating the mercury myth who hates people with autism and wants to "cure" them*. What in the hell was I thinking?

That I wanted to tell an important story, he reminded me. That thousands upon thousands of parents are living this exact same story. They may be facing different versions of regression and recovery, maybe different acronyms—ADHD, ASD, SPD, and so forth—but what we lived through and what they are living through is *real*.

And maybe instead of beating myself up so badly about what I did or didn't do, I needed to remember this: three hospitals, four pediatricians, three neurologists, one ear, nose, and throat specialist, one entire surgical staff, two sets of emergency room staff, four speech therapists, two early intervention specialists, and the entire team of specialists in the school all missed it.

For four years, not one of them thought to run a urine test to check for toxins; to consider that maybe we were being overprescribed medication and antibiotics; to send me to a developmental pediatrician; or to *listen* to me.

And when it was finally proven I was right, it was suggested we might not be a good fit for their practice anymore because we didn't want to take any chances with our youngest child, who happened to get her first ear infection at the exact same age as her sister and whom we decided to stop vaccinating until we knew for absolutely certain the same thing wouldn't happen to her. They even made us sign a humiliating document stating we were basically bad parents for doing so.

Don't you dare blame yourself, he told me. We were the ones let down by the system. We were the ones beat up and abused by it. We still are. And we made it anyway. Our position is reasonable, it's responsible, and it's not without merit. The way we have been treated is deplorable. We have nothing to be ashamed of, he insisted.

And so after a few days, I finally got the stomach to agree. It doesn't matter what anyone else thinks or believes about what happened to our daughter anyway. It only matters what we believe. And we chose not to believe it was a coincidence.

Autism and all that surrounds its symptoms, its onset, its recovery, its explosion, its ratio of boys to girls, its history, its biology, its science, its politics, and so much more is supposedly nothing more than an unfortunate coincidence, the experts claim.

Clearly, I can't change their minds. I wish I could. At the very least, I can be grateful that I changed mine and was able to challenge the existing assumptions. In doing so, I finally got the answers to two very important questions.

One, it turns out Emma's favorite color is actually purple.

And two, elephants eat grass because they are herbivores that require a large amount of readily available food, such as grasses, tree bark, and other vegetation.

ACKNOWLEDGMENTS

I'd like to thank everyone who has always believed in me, not only as a mother, family member, colleague, and friend, but also as a writer. To my parents, who bought me my first typewriter for eighth-grade graduation; to my grandmother, who kept every single thing I ever wrote and always encouraged me to continue; to Dan Olmsted and Mark Blaxill, who gave me my first formal opportunity; to David Kirby, who once told me I was gifted (maybe the highest compliment I have ever received and why I believed I could do this); to Lou Conte and Tony Lyons, my dear friends at Skyhorse Publishing, who made this possible; and to all of my readers, who have let me know how much they appreciate what I write. Thank you. I hope I told our story well.

Also, to my editor, thank you for your unending patience and guidance. This is one of the hardest things I have ever done.

To my parents, thank you for everything, just everything. I could have never survived or done any of this without you.

Dad, you gave me the gift of analysis and the example of what it means to have integrity. You taught me what it means to stand up for something even when you are standing alone. You taught me to trust logic and myself. And you taught me you could (and should) still laugh, have fun, and have a great life even when you are taking on the world. Thank you.

Mom, you are the strongest woman I have ever known. You taught me to confront life head on, to never tolerate bullshit, and to be wise beyond my years. Your love and wisdom have made me the woman I am and will guide me to be the amazing woman I have yet to become. Thank you for always being there.

To both of you, your faith in your granddaughter and me, your support for us, and your love for us got me through my darkest days. The same is true for my in-laws, the most generous, loving, accepting people I have ever met. Thank you. I love you more than words can express.

To my brothers, in-laws, cousins, aunts, uncles, and extended family on both sides that have also always supported us, too, thank you. And to my guardian angels, who I know are keeping watch over us, Grandma, Grandma-Grandma, and Aunt Gail, I thank you and miss you every day.

To my cousin, Meredith, for having the courage to say what everyone wanted to, but didn't know how. Thank you.

To my best friends, Kristen, Kristin, Gina, Angela, and Renee, the extended family I have been blessed with since childhood, I don't know how I would have survived this without you, either. Your friendship, love, and laughter are some of the greatest gifts in my life. Thank you for supporting me, tolerating me, and never giving up on me.

To my very best friend, Allison, for all of that and so much more . . . thank you. No one has ridden this roller coaster more with me than you.

To Karen, Jay, Jane, Tim, Suzanne, Dave, and Kate, thank you for your continued friendship and support. Karen and Jay, thank you for always including us in your lives, for sharing our heartbreak and frustration, and for setting the bar for what it means to be great parents; Jane and Tim, thank you for being our best friends and the best neighbors possible, and for always loving us through the good times and bad; Dave and Suzanne, thank you for always giving us a great time and including us too; and Kate, thank you for always being there and hearing me out even when we didn't always agree.

To all of the families and friends of the children in our community and elsewhere who have always welcomed our daughter into your lives, including her and looking out for her, even when you didn't have to, thank you.

Jackie, Joan, Jill, Janet, and Helen, your love and concern for our daughter have not gone unnoticed or unappreciated. Emma, Hannah, and Talia the same. Thank you. I cannot possibly put into words what it means.

To my colleagues over the years, especially those who always listened to my endless discussions about my daughter and autism, especially Barb, Clare, Brigit, and Maggie, and to everyone else I shared a school with who always supported my choices and my career no matter what, thank you. I miss you.

To all of the teachers, aides, bus drivers, faculty, and staff in our school district who have always had our daughter's best interest at heart, thank you.

To Brandan, the best case-manager I've ever known, the same. Autism is hard enough without worrying your child isn't safe at school. Thank you for always giving us the peace of mind of knowing she was not only safe, but loved.

To my entire extended circle of friends, family, childhood friends, and community members on Facebook who have never blocked or unfriended me in spite of my passionate and endless posts. I can't believe it. Thank you!

To my fellow parents, advocates, and activists who have become my extended family and best friends in the search for truth and healing, too many of you to list. You know who you are. I can't imagine my life without you. You are the strongest, most courageous, most intelligent, inspiring, badass group of people I have ever met. I'm honored to call you all friends. Thank you.

To Mary Holland and Kim Mack Rosenberg for your friendship, intelligence, and helping me edit, thank you.

To Kevin Barry and Becky Estepp, two of my closest friends and two of the fiercest advocates on earth. I love you both, and I thank you for your never-ending love and support.

To Dan Olmsted and Mark Blaxill, for believing in me, and for never giving up on the truth. Thank you.

To Eric Gladen, for giving up your life to tell a story you didn't have to. Thank you for your dedication to the cause and for including me in it.

To Bobby Kennedy, for allowing me a glimpse into your life, and for everything you have done to bring this tragic episode of American history and injustice to an end. My family is forever indebted. Thank you.

To J. B. and Lisa Handley, for having the courage to start Generation Rescue; to Jenny McCarthy, for being the bravest, most courageous celebrity on the planet, and taking this amazing organization over; to Candace McDonald, for having the vision and ability to make it what it is; and to Peter and Michelle Doyle, for including us in your pursuit of helping affected families. Thank you, all.

To all of the doctors, scientists, therapists, and practitioners who dedicate their lives to helping and healing children on the spectrum, thank you.

To all of the legislators, journalists, bloggers, and celebrities dedicated to the truth as well, thank you, too.

And finally, to my E., my M., my M., and my A. You are the reason any of this was possible and my reason for doing it. You are my light, my love, and my soft place to fall. I love you all with every ounce of my being. Thank you for loving me in return.

But most especially, to my E., the greatest teacher I have ever had . . . an angel on earth, here to show us the error of our ways . . . a beautiful canary in the coal mine.

I will never be able to tell you how sorry I am, Sweetie. I will never be able to go back and make it right. But I can tell you this.

It matters what happened to you, E. You mattered. You still matter. All of the children like you matter. And I will make sure of it for the rest of my life.